Biomechanics

of

Human

Communication

BIOMECHANICS
OF
HUMAN
COMMUNICATION

Neurophysiology, Regulation, and Systems Thinking

STEFANIE FAYE MOLICKI

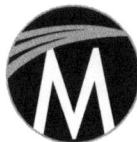

MERCURY LEARNING AND INFORMATION
Boston, Massachusetts

Publisher: David Pallai
MERCURY LEARNING AND INFORMATION
121 High Street, 3rd Floor
Boston, MA 02110
info@merclearning.com
www.merclearning.com
800-232-0223

S. Faye Molicki. *Biomechanics of Human Communication: Neurophysiology, Regulation, and Systems Thinking*
ISBN: 978-1-68392-922-2

Library of Congress Control Number: 2023945503

232425321   This book is printed on acid-free paper in the United States of America.

CONTENTS

Preface   xi

Acknowledgments   xv

**CHAPTER 1: SYSTEMS, FEEDBACK, AND
             EXPERIENCE-DEPENDENCE: A LOOK AT
             COMPLEXITY AND HUMAN BRAIN
             DEVELOPMENT**   1

Systems Thinking   4

Experience Dependence   9

Attachment Experiences and Brain Development   12

    Off-Loading and Outsourcing   14

    Serve and Return Feedback   15

Feedback as a Tool for Regulating Nervous Systems   18

    Contingent Responsivity   19

Locomotion Changes the Communication Patterns of the
  Caregiver-Child Relationship   20

    Social Referencing   20

Summary   23

References   23

**CHAPTER 2: SIGNAL DISTORTION: UNCONSCIOUS FILTERS
        THAT BIAS COMMUNICATION AND PERCEPTION   29**

Regulatory Flexibility   30

   Context Sensitivity   32

   Context Insensitivity   32

   Repertoire   33

   Feedback   34

      Internal Feedback   34

      Social Feedback   36

   Feedback Responsiveness   36

Challenges to Regulatory Flexibility   37

   Implicit and Procedural Memory   38

   The Orbital Prefrontal Cortex and Procedural Memory   39

   Anticipation and Preparation   41

Feedback, Stress Regulation, and Autonomic Responses   41

   Inescapability   44

   Repetitive Exposure   45

   Predictive Biases   45

   Limited Data Means Less Accurate Algorithms   48

Chapter Summary   50

References   51

**CHAPTER 3: COMMUNICATION AS A FORM OF FEEDBACK
        RESPONSIVENESS, BIOBEHAVIORAL
        ATTUNEMENT, AND ATTACHMENT   61**

Attachment Theory Is in Fact "Regulation Theory"   64

   So What Is Attachment Theory?   64

   Secure and Insecure Attachment   65

Effective Communication Is an Ongoing Process of
Feedback Responsiveness   65

   Biobehavioral Synchrony: An Emphasis on Bottom-Up,
      Clearly Observable Patterns   66

   Autonomic Reactivity and Vagal Tone   68

Affiliative Hormones and Brain Activation 69

Oxytocin and Gender 71

Lack of Biobehavioral Synchrony 71

High-Risk Parenting 73

Other Factors That Can Influence Biobehavioral Patterns 74

Chapter Summary 74

References 75

CHAPTER 4: COMMUNICATION AS A BEHAVIORAL TRANSMITTER AND ENERGY OPTIMIZER **79**

Communication for Survival 80

Communication is a Warning Signal to Attempt to Prevent the Physical Proximity of a Threat or Predator 82

Communication is an Airborne Signal to Request Help or Support in the Case of Illness, Distress, or Injury 82

Communication to Organize Behavior Against a Threat 83

Communication for Energy Optimization 84

Human Optimization Through Sociality 86

Communication as a Sociobehavioral Transmitter 87

Modern Attachment Theory 88

Dynamic-Maturational Model of Attachment and Adaptation 89

Danger, Adaptation, and Maladaptation: An Information Processing Model of Attachment 90

SHORTCUTS 91

Protective Strategies: Overview of DMM Categories 94

Chapter Summary 97

References 98

CHAPTER 5: THE MECHANICS OF COMMUNICATION SIGNALS **101**

Direct Contact Communication Versus Telereception 102

Voluntary Versus Involuntary Systems 102

Eyes, Voice, and Face 104

The Role of Eyes in Communication 104

Pupil Dilation   104

Eye Gaze   105

The Role of Facial Expressions in Communication   106

The Component Process Model of Emotion (CPM)   107

Embodied Cognition and Emotion Expression   111

The Effects of Trauma on Emotional Facial Expression   112

Summary   114

References   115

CHAPTER 6: COMMUNICATION AND THE VOICE-HEART
CONNECTION   **121**

Voice and Communication   122

The Voice-Face-Heart Connection   122

Human Voice Mechanisms and Features   125

The Physiological Basis of Vocalizing   125

Source-Filter Theory   126

Speech Production   131

Voice Features and Affective State   131

Voice Features and Mental Health   132

How Stress Affects Voice   132

Depression and Voice   134

Suicidality and Voice   135

Post-traumatic Stress and Voice   136

Anger and Voice   136

Sleep Deprivation and Voice   136

Information Contained in the Voice   136

The Brunswikian Functional Lens Model   137

Perceiving Voice   140

Sound Frequencies and Nervous System Responses   141

Physiology of the Middle Ear   142

Perception of Voices and Mental Health   145

Vocal Expressions of Positive Emotions   146

Summary   146

References   147

CHAPTER 7: SOCIAL COMMUNICATION: HOW NONVERBAL AND VERBAL ELEMENTS CONVERGE AND ENHANCE OUR COMMUNICATION ABILITIES   161

Social Communication   162

Social Communication and Executive Functioning   162

Social Communication and Social Synchrony   163

Social Communication and Joint Attention   163

Social Communication and Theory of Mind   164

Nonverbal and Verbal Components of Social Communication   165

Language as a Bridge   165

Using Words to Describe Emotion: Emotional Granularity   166

Alexithymia and Challenges in Describing Emotions   167

Cognitive, Emotional, and Linguistic Aspects of Alexithymia   168

Prioritization of Emotional Cues in Verbal and Nonverbal Communication   170

Lateralization   172

Faster Processing of Nonverbal Emotional Vocalizations   172

Perception of Emotional Written Words   173

Perception of Emotional Spoken Words   174

Summary   176

References   177

CHAPTER 8: THE ROLE OF MATURITY, EXECUTIVE FUNCTIONING, AND SOCIAL UNDERSTANDING IN COMMUNICATION   195

The Complexity of Social Understanding   196

Social Understanding and Language   197

Language as a Cognitive Niche and Psychological Tool   198

Private and Inner Speech   199

Cognitive Flexibility and Communication   201

Cognitive Processes and Distortions   201

Relational Frame Theory   202

Relational Frame Theory and the Lang Fear Network   202

Cognitive Therapies   205

Generic Versus Nongeneric Language   205

Self-Disclosure and Attributions   207

Summary   208

References   208

CHAPTER 9: SYSTEMS RESILIENCE   **215**

Resilience and Survivability   216

What Makes a System Resilient?   219

Passive and Active Resilience   220

Protection   221

Rupture, Repair, and Flexible Responsiveness   224

Assets   226

Quality Attributes of Resilience   228

Guiding Principles for Resilient Systems   229

Chapter Summary   232

Book Summary   232

References   237

INDEX   **241**

PREFACE

The first time I experienced a lie detector test, my worldview changed forever. I was sitting in a hotel room, hooked up to metal plates. Electrodes and sensors all over my face, body, straps around my chest. Every twitch, every fluctuation would be measured as I answered questions. I had been hired by a government agency and this was the final step in getting my security clearance.

There's no way a machine can tell if I'm lying, I remember thinking. I would soon be proven wrong. To establish a baseline of what my nervous system would do during a lie, the examiner created a scenario where I had to lie. So I did. As I spoke the words of this untruth (it had to do with a deck of cards, so nothing too emotional or deep), I didn't feel a change in my response. I couldn't tell any difference whatsoever between when I answered the questions truthfully or untruthfully. In fact, after that line of questioning, I started to wonder - what if there is no difference? What would that say about me? That I'm comfortable being dishonest? Maybe somehow that's a good thing for this job? Would being good at lying make me a bad person?

I soon got my answer. Once all the sensors were removed and we discussed the test, I was shown, on multiple monitors, what my body's physiological response was to telling falsehoods. In frames showing my deceptive answer, every single measurement had skyrocketed - off the chart, literally. I was shocked. How could I not have noticed all of those changes that clearly shifted so significantly from my baseline that they couldn't even be captured on the same graph?

That was my first introduction to the world of frequencies and signals. Vibrations that we transmit, and that are observable and detectable by something outside of us. Without being able to go into more detail about what I did during that chapter of my career, I can say that I learned, from a meta-perspective, what signals and communication patterns can reveal about human behavior, information-sharing and predictability.

My next encounter with human-based frequencies would be years later, in a neuroscience lab at New York University. I was a graduate student, assisting a postdoc, with studies on disgust, moral decision-making and stereotypes. I studied and reported on changes in electric conductance of skin (galvanic skin response), facial electromyography and heart rate variability. Alongside all of this neurophysiological data, I also helped conduct studies on social emotional learning and attachment with the NYU Institute for Prevention Studies and Yeshiva University's College of Medicine. In my fieldwork, I conducted interviews and experimental vignettes with kids, implemented reading and social emotional interventions, and coded interview data from parents. All of those experiences have helped inform much of the work I do today in the field of neuropsychology.

The concept of communication is complex. How people communicate with each other has powerful consequences for human behavior, mental health and overall performance. My goal with this book is to help people become more aware of all the ways we express and receive communication signals that are influenced by many forces beyond our awareness. Translating these experiences into words on a page helps us observe them, recognize patterns and hopefully illuminate ways for us to use communication as a tool for true understanding, healing and connection.

The other purpose of this book is to create a neurophysiology-based framework for assessing and improving communication. It introduces measurable and neurobiologically-informed concepts and language to help increase awareness of what factors may be influencing communicative interactions. Through this, it is my hope that we may - whether as professionals helping clients or as individuals interacting with people in our daily life - learn how to use communication in ways that promote resilience, adaptability and understanding.

The Core Proposition

This book is an exploration of human communication patterns through the lens of neurophysiology, systems thinking, and attachment frameworks. It is an investigation into the biomechanical and vibrational-based nature of social communication and how the flow of information from one person to another and from one internal system to another can powerfully influence the brain's and nervous system's ability to adapt to challenges and create social connection.

From Brain Development to Systems Resilience

This book begins with foundational concepts related to brain development, including experience-dependent neuroplasticity and frameworks for understanding how complex organisms respond to stimulus. It then guides the reader across multiple frameworks and theories that inform our understanding of how and why humans communicate, and what causes distortions and challenges in communication. Later chapters explore the biomechanical systems that enable human communication, and how these communication systems affect human brain development and nervous system regulation. The book concludes with a look at how communication tools and strategies play a role in the resilience of systems that include individuals, relationships and communities.

Global Audience

This book is designed for a wide audience. The language used is geared for people with some basic knowledge of human psychology and behavior, but is intended for people who are beginners in their understanding of neuroscience, as well as professionals who are very familiar with the field of neuropsychology and want to deepen their understanding of the biomechanical side of communication, emotion regulation and attachment theory. Although there are technical terms used throughout the book, they are explained at a level that is meant for non-technical and general audiences.

Stefanie Faye Molicki
October 2023

ACKNOWLEDGMENTS

I would like to acknowledge all the researchers who dedicate their time and energy to helping us better understand the experience of being human. And to all the guides, teachers, partners, friends and companions who help us get in touch with wisdom that leads us to live our lives more fully, authentically and lovingly - and that we would not get to on our own.

SYSTEMS, FEEDBACK, AND EXPERIENCE-DEPENDENCE: A LOOK AT COMPLEXITY AND HUMAN BRAIN DEVELOPMENT

Why do some conversations end up in arguments while others help us find solutions? How do we get better at saying what we truly want to say? What are we trying to do when we communicate with others? Communication is at the heart of our social existence. It can soothe, innovate, mediate, and escalate behaviors and nervous system states. It can bring people closer together and cultivate understanding. It can also push people apart, leaving them feeling more misunderstood than when they tried to engage in dialogue. Communication is a vast and complex topic. At its most basic level, we can understand it as exchanging information through signs, symbols, and behaviors. This type of definition, however, lacks the diversity of layers that go into each moment of human communication. As we will see throughout this book, communication is an aspect of human experience that reflects our personal and collective histories, what we have been exposed to regarding social interactions, and what may have been neglected. Exploring communication allows us to understand human interaction more deeply: it conveys our internal states and intentions, what we perceive as our values and goals, and what we can cope with. It examines emotions, feelings, senses, computations, cognitions, distortions, and social systems. This book will regularly return to complexity and systems thinking as a foundation for understanding the various communication layers, including nervous systems, social and family systems, and concepts from systems engineering and resilience. Our exploration of communication from this perspective will lead us to important questions we will attempt to answer while leaving space for more sophisticated curiosities and future pathways.

For example, when we say communication is a tool for exchanging information, what information is being exchanged? Second, how is this done—what are these common symbols, signs, and behaviors? Third, is that all communication is for? Is it only for exchanging information, or are there other purposes? In other words, why are we communicating? And fourth, does our process of communication achieve its goal? If it is a process of exchanging information, does it accomplish this? If there are other purposes, are those achieved? This book is an attempt to provoke thought about these ideas and questions as a way to help us not only understand but also to refine and hone our use of communication as a tool to enhance and evolve our intelligence, relationships, and sense of well-being. As we will uncover in upcoming sections, human communication dynamics have long histories embedded in each moment. Understanding and navigating the complexity of human communication requires us to think not only about the mechanisms we use but also about what we are trying to do when we communicate.

It is helpful to consider how other species send signals and exchange information to expand our ideas about how and why humans communicate. Nonhuman species have a variety of mechanisms for communication. Insects, for example, use antenna-tapping, dancing (such as bees to indicate a nectar source), chemicals (such as pheromones), sound vibrations, and visual cues, such as patterns and colors [NC2022]. Aquatic creatures primarily use sound waves [DOSITS2022]. Land mammals, birds, nonhuman primates, and humans create vibrations that travel through the air for others to sense. In this book, we will focus on human communication, particularly the beats that others can see and hear (audible and visible signals), which includes facial gestures, vocalizations (sounds and words), graphical representations (written or illustrated words and symbols), and body and limb movements (such as fist clenching, eye movement, posture, etc.). We create these audible and visible signals by using muscles to move bones. We move muscles in our face, throat, diaphragm, ears, limbs, and body to create a mechanical output of an internal experience. These movements develop vibrations that disrupt air molecules as they leave the body. As these molecules bump up against each other, they create waves that travel across the air and can be detected by various sensory receptors of another organism.

Air
Molecules

Amplitude

|← Wavelength →|

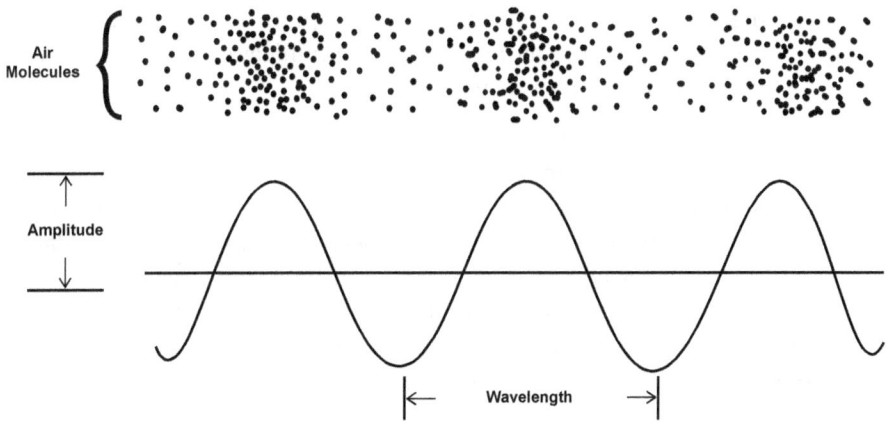

The vibrations we create through these movements are the biomechanical transmissions of communication. These are the signals and frequencies we transmit and receive during our interactions. These movements and vibrations do not occur in a vacuum. Multiple systems influence each other to create the fluctuations of frequencies we use to communicate. Understanding how and why these movements occur plays a significant role in understanding communication patterns. There are a variety of reasons that we will explore in coming sections and chapters:

- The vibrations we transmit are influenced by our internal state. Our inner condition affects mechanisms such as our breath, facial microexpressions, limb movement and posture, and configurations of our pharyngeal and laryngeal muscles and other mechanisms to convey voice frequencies.

- Our internal state carries with it many implicit and autonomic processes that are below our awareness. Many of these unconscious aspects of our inner state affect what we communicate to others without understanding.

- Our earliest experiences with communication and social interaction highly influenced these processes. These processes influence how we perceive and interpret stimuli from others and the external world.

- Suppose we have challenges in regulating our internal state. In that case, we may end up transmitting and detecting signals that lead to a distortion in communication (such as perceiving a threat when it is not present and then displaying defensive behaviors).

- If we are not aware that these unconscious processes are occurring, we may continue to repeat patterns of communication without recognizing there are repeating patterns. A repetitive pattern indicates a lack of flexibility, which may mean the communication is not responding adaptively to emergent information.

As we can see from the above points, we must include the complexity of our histories and unconscious influences to understand human communication. A word or facial gesture will lead to a different response for each person based on their internal state and what they become aware of—both related to their past experiences and current neural and behavioral resources. No universal vibration or symbol of communication will cause the same effect in every human being; too many other factors come into play. Regarding this type of complexity, a systems-thinking mindset can be helpful.

SYSTEMS THINKING

A problem never exists on its own. As systems theorist Russell Ackoff asserts, problems are constantly surrounded by other problems in space and time. The more we can expand our view of the complex web of interactions and systems surrounding a problem, the more chance we have of finding an adequate solution [ACKOFF1978]. Other problems cover any challenges we have in our communication abilities and cause–effect relationships that we may not consider during an interaction. Expanding our view of where ineffective communication may be linked with and influenced by other challenges and causes is a fundamental aspect of systems thinking. Systems thinking is about shifting, widening, and deepening how we look at the world. It is an ability to zoom out as wide as possible to see interconnected nodes and how they interact and then to zoom back in to re-examine a problem in a new light while still holding that wider perspective. It is a paradigm—a way of looking at the world—through many lenses and perspectives. These perspectives also consider the histories and multiple systems nested in other systems that may influence the behavior of what we are looking at. When trying to understand a system, especially a complex system such as a brain, a person, a family, a community, or a communication system, we cannot look at one individual node or part in isolation. To truly understand it, we must explore how that system interacts with other systems and nodes. This is the case when we talk about a person's nervous system, mental health, brain, and communication patterns. None of these occur in isolation. The responses and signals within an interaction happen about everything that each person has experienced until that point and are related to all the other nervous systems and environments they are currently interacting with.

Therefore, we cannot use a linear approach to understand what is occurring during communication. This means we cannot predict that a word or facial gesture will universally induce the same response. Each interaction between people as they communicate is *emergent*. Emergence reflects the idea that as each person sends signals out, the other person reacts to those, changing the subsequent reaction of the other. Both unconscious and conscious processes influence each person's responses. These processes are built through the historical data each person has accumulated before that interaction. Each person's individual history-based predictions and computations then interact with the data that emerges continuously during the exchange. For this reason, expanding our view of what occurs across time and space can help us understand communication.

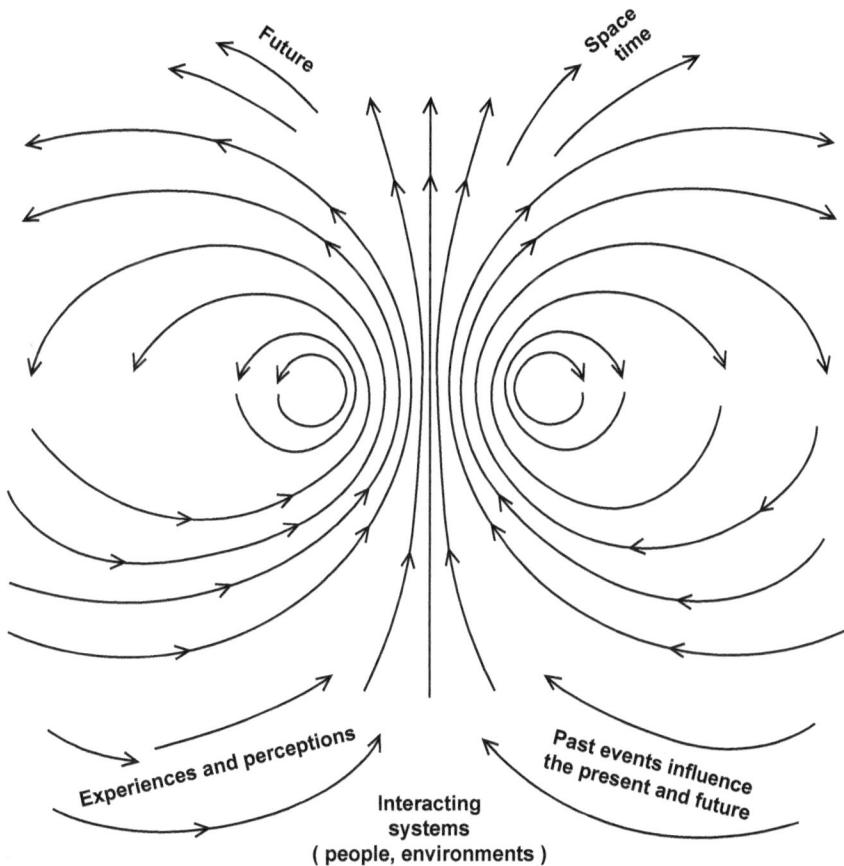

Future

Space time

Experiences and perceptions

Past events influence the present and future

Interacting
systems
(people, environments)

Expanding our view of time and space to see histories and multiple interacting nodes and systems to study behavior is part of the paradigm of systems thinking.

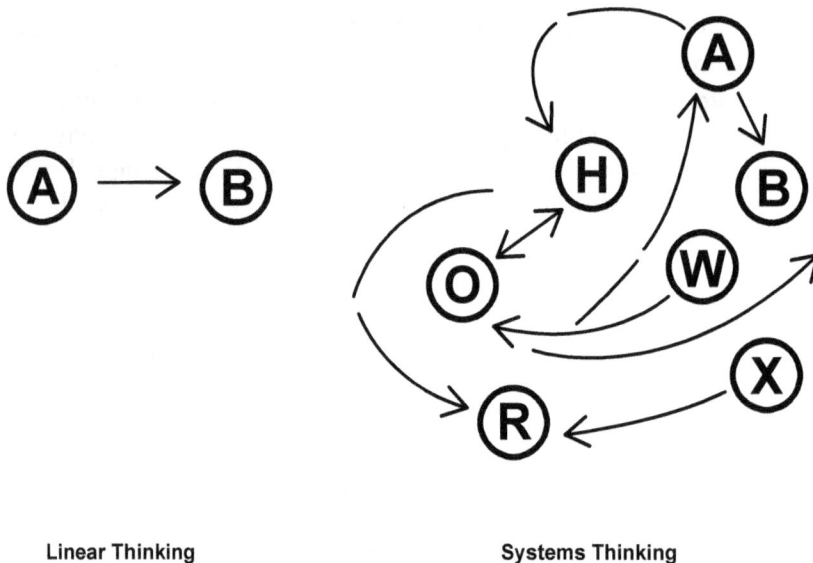

Linear Thinking   **Systems Thinking**

Systems thinking is in contrast to linear or simple cause–effect reasoning. One of these cause–effect models is stimulus–response. The stimulus–response paradigm is the idea that the stimulus causes a response, and nothing mediates this response between those stages.

We can observe this direct, one-to-one stimulus–response reaction in certain organisms:

- Irritability: This describes the response that occurs in the cell fluid of single-celled organisms in direct response to a change in environment [ERULKAR2023].

- Taxis: In simple organisms, such as algae and fungi, taxis describe the response to move toward or away from the stimuli [ZUG2022].

A major contributor to the stimulus–response model was the law of effect, which stated that if a behavioral response (R) resulted in a satisfactory result, this would increase the chance that the behavioral response would continue to reoccur in response to the stimulus (S) [RAFFERTY2023]. This premise underlies the idea of conditioning, which became a significant part of psychological and physiological research in the early 1900s. Through this simple cause–effect (stimulus–response) framework, a stimulus (such as an electric shock or something rewarding, such as food) is given to elicit a response.

A term we can use to describe the basic S–R model is *unmediated*. There is no in-between process or mediator between the stimulus and the response. If we were to try to apply the S–R model to more complex organisms, we would see that something is missing in the equation. For example, if a traumatic event such as a natural disaster occurs (stimulus), according to the S–R model, we can reliably predict a person's response. If an event such as winning the lottery occurs, we would also more or less be able to predict the response because, according to this model, the *event* or stimulus directly *causes* the response. As we can see from the above two examples, and as research has demonstrated, humans do not have a universal response to winning the lottery or tragic events [BRICKMAN1978; BONANNO2013]. The event does not have a simple, direct link to the response.

From an energy-conservation perspective, it makes sense that we often try to find the simplest cause–effect explanation. Without a mediating factor, we could more easily predict and control outcomes. In that sense, we may tend to seek out simple cause–effect relationships so that we can better predict our world. As Langhe and colleagues reflect in their article "Linear Thinking in a Nonlinear World," although people have a tendency to expect direct, linear relationships, links between variables and outcomes are frequently not linear[LANGHE2017]. The challenge is that, without realizing it, we may be trying to understand our own behaviors or the behaviors of others through this type of simple cause–effect relationship. And as you can likely guess, human behavior is not this simple.

While it is possible that certain stimuli (such as an electric shock) could lead to fairly predictable responses in humans, the complexity and experience-dependent nature of the human nervous system (which we will explore in the next section) adds a complex, emergent, and dynamic factor to the equation. Because of this complexity, a simple cause–effect model such as stimulus–response is generally insufficient for understanding and predicting human behavior and communication. Complex adaptive organisms such as humans have multiple systems that synchronize and integrate events. A stimulus does not interact with just one part of you. Various systems are working together within you, and each responds to conditions in their own way that contributes to the entire organization of your response.

For example, in response to a sound, such as a voice or a bang, it is not just your ear that receives this stimulus and then responds. Vibrations from the sound also hit your skin and bones. The sensory receptors throughout your body receive information in different ways. In response to the vibrational patterns that hit these sensors, some of your subsystems will receive more oxygen and blood flow while others receive less. While the types of responses may vary, the interactions are organized. Each subsystem does not act on its own without communication from other systems. Your left leg does not move in its own direction without any coordination of what the rest of the body is doing. Your pupils do not constrict or dilate without some communication flow with other parts of your body. Control mechanisms help coordinate, synchronize, and integrate what your body's parts and systems do together in response to something. These mechanisms occur in *between* stimulus and response. This means the formula is not S–R. There is something that mediates the relationship. That mediator is the organism—a complex, dynamic system with a history.

This paradigm is the Stimulus–Organism–Response model [WOODWORTH1918]. It acknowledges that there is a mediating factor between stimulus and response. A person's response to a stimulus can be mediated and moderated by various highly interrelated factors:

- Current neurochemical activity may be influenced by things such as how much they have slept, what they have eaten, immune system functioning, temperature of the environment, etc.

- Their neural and behavioral resources (the circuitries, brain activation patterns, and behavioral repertoires that are most accessible at a given moment).

- Their past experiences may lead to sensitivities and anticipatory adjustments [PAYNE2015].

- How they interpret information and create narratives and explanations about events, which may be influenced by sociocultural factors and past events.

We must keep in mind that the organism in the S–O–R model constantly interacts with other systems and has a long history of interactions that influence their perceptions and behaviors, brain development, and communication patterns. We see this paradigm reflected particularly in the study of holobionts. The holobiont paradigm in biology is the understanding that an organism is not understandable in isolation. The systems, environments, and organisms that live in, on, and around it are all part of a dynamic field of interaction [BAEDKE2020]. Throughout this book, we will continue to see that communication is intimately connected to multiple overlapping systems, including our ability to regulate our nervous system, which is deeply influenced by our social, relational, and family systems and past and present experiences. Therefore, human brain development and the resulting communication behaviors are "experience-dependent."

EXPERIENCE DEPENDENCE

While the brain's development is highly influenced by genetic factors, vast amounts and features of the brain are entirely dependent on what a person is exposed to regarding social and environmental stimuli [HARVARDDC1]. In particular, the brain's frontal cortex takes years to develop and is one of the last to mature, making it the least constrained by genes and the most shaped and influenced by experience [SAPOLSKY2017]. This dependence on experience rather than predetermination by genetic programming, particularly for the sophisticated potentials of the frontal brain areas, gives the human species incredible flexibility and adaptability [SAPOLSKY2017, TEGMARK2017]. Another related term is experience-expectant development, which refers to a process where experiences that occur during a very narrow period early on in life significantly impact subsequent development [NELSON2014]. These can include experiences with patterned light that helps with visual development and experiences with faces and speech that help language and communication development. In contrast, experience-dependent development continues and can be shaped throughout the lifespan [NELSON2014]. While we will discuss very early experiences that align with experience-expectant development, we will focus on experience-dependent processes that occur from birth onwards.

To help us understand the concept of experience–expectant and experience–dependent brain development, it can be helpful to look at what happens when experiences are significantly outside of the norm, such as in cases of severe neglect and deprivation. Neuroscience researchers captured some of these dramatic effects by studying the brain of a specific group of orphans. In the late 1980s, at the fall of Romanian dictator Nicolae Ceausescu's regime, many children in Romania who had been orphaned or unable to be cared for adequately during the war were placed in orphanages. Due to a lack of government funding to repay the debt, the orphanages' electricity and food were intermittent, and space and personnel were limited [NELSON2014].

The children were placed in metal cribs, all adjacent to each other. They were rarely touched, held, spoken to, or played with. Many stayed in the cribs even as they got older until age 5, 6, or 7. Abuse, neglect, corporal punishment, and unsanitary conditions were common [NELSON2014].

When the war ended, orphanages were opened to aid workers and researchers. One of these researchers, Charles Nelson from Harvard Medical School, noticed odd behaviors, delayed language, and other symptoms suggesting brain development problems [NELSON2019]. He and other researchers began studying the children using electroencephalography (EEG), which measures electrical activity in the brain [VANDERWERT2010]. As the children grew older, they could use magnetic resonance imaging to study their brains. They found that many of the orphans had significantly lower brain activity levels than other children. Another disturbing result was that their brains were physically smaller, dramatically reducing gray and white matter [FOX2010]. The researchers discovered this was not merely a malnutrition or poor physical condition. What was becoming clear was that the problems in brain development were related to lack of attachment to a caregiver, or "psychosocial deprivation" [NELSON2019]. This brings us to a few important points worth explaining about the brain.[1]

First, why would a brain be smaller due to neglect? In other words, what about stimulation and enriching environments make a brain "big?" One aspect of this involves the folds of the brain—the wrinkles and crevices (also known as sulci or sulcus for singular). The folds and wrinkles are nature's way of increasing the number of connections and information-sharing materials inside the fixed size of the skull. If our skills continuously grew with more information we gathered from conception and throughout our lives, we would have giant heads. This may not sound like a bad thing, except that our neck muscles, joints, spine, and skeleton would also have to grow proportionately to keep up with holding ourselves upright. Since information-sharing continues to activate new circuits, the process is ongoing, which means head and body size would need to grow to contain the brain continually. Instead of continually needing to make things bigger, one of nature's solutions is to increase surface area by introducing extra edges.[2] For example, the tiny hairs all over

---

[1] In this section, we will look at brain development in a general way; in Chapter 2, we will look at a particular area of the frontal cortex that is impacted by experiences, particularly psychosocial conditions.

[2] Another strategy is "off-loading" or "out-sourcing" which we will look at later in this chapter.

and inside our body, like the leaves and branches on trees, are nature's way of increasing surface area without continuously expanding the entire structure. The wrinkles and crevices within the brain are another way this occurs. As exposure to feedback and data increases, the brain-body vehicle must process more information. This requires neurons, glial cells, interneurons, and many more types of material that act as nodes, connectors, and other network-building mechanisms [KOLK22]. All complex adaptive systems have ways of sharing information through nodes and connectors. More information means more materials are needed to connect and share it.

A city can be used to illustrate this. Just like the brain, a city is also a complex adaptive system. Nodes are the people, buildings, etc. Roadways and communication infrastructure are connective structures. Signals are transmitted in many ways across all of the structures. If the city grows in population, more signals are being transmitted and received, so more material is needed to accommodate this. More grocery stores, cell phone towers, and roadways that are either higher in number or larger in size. Suppose the city's boundaries are more or less established politically or because of landscape limitations such as being surrounded by water or mountains. In that case, the material becomes denser, and there are often higher edges and crevices (think skyscrapers and elevated transit systems or roadways). Contrast this to a quiet town in the middle of a geographically isolated region. There are likely no skyscrapers, and the buildings can be relatively low and spread out. Fewer communication signals are being exchanged at every moment. If the city never needed to interact with another city to survive, fewer nodes and connections would be adequate for self-sustaining. To a certain degree, it could maintain its own homeostasis by extracting resources from its environment. The nature and size of the city may not become dramatically larger as time goes by if it is not interacting with many other cities or sources of information.

The difference between a small town and a human brain is that a small town can stay geographically immobile and create self-organizing systems within that stable location. Moreover, a city or town comprises humans who move from one location to the next and interact with other humans. The ability to locomote and interact socially enables us to access a higher number and a higher variety of resources to maintain homeostasis. This locomotive ability plays a large role in our brain development and intelligence (which we explore even further in this chapter). Locomotion and movement mean that we cross many different terrains and situations where we must engage in problem-solving and decision-making. It also means we cross many different social dynamics, hierarchies, and systems within our lifetime. The emergent and unpredictable challenges and opportunities within the environment require an ongoing ability to adapt to new movements and behaviors. This high level of adaptability can be achieved by using experiences to build movement patterns and internal working models for responding to the unique set of conditions that a human is exposed to from birth. As the brain responds to stimulating and enriching environments, it continues to increase the complexity of its networks [KEMPERMANN2019]. This requires network-building material and, therefore, more cells and connective resources in the brain, increasing gray and white matter.

Consequently, if a child is born into an environment with little challenge or interaction with a variety of people and experiences, the brain lacks the stimulation it needs to create new connections and circuits [NSCDC2012]. This would result in smaller size and impairments in overall functioning [NSCDC2012]. In addition to allowing more flexibility for continuous growth, experience-dependent brain-building is also nature's way of using energy more efficiently. Suppose energy is being used to activate and build systems that are not being used. In that case, that energy is unavailable to maintain, repair, and build other resources that are being asked for by the environment. From a systems perspective, it is more efficient to use resources for current situational requirements and "get rid of" structures that are not being used so that they no longer tie up energy. This is referred to as pruning [KOLK2022; HARVARDDC1]. As we leave the womb, the cortex responds with an explosion of activity and neuronal overgrowth and then prunes this overgrowth away as the infant interacts with its environment [KOLK2022; HARVARDDC1]. To sum up, we do not have all of the networks and architecture preprogrammed from birth to guide *all* of our behavior for the rest of our lives. Instead, a significant amount of networks and connections are formed based on the exposure to experiences unique to each individual. The brain depends on genes to lay a foundation, but it depends on experiences to modify and build much of its architecture [FOX2010].

ATTACHMENT EXPERIENCES AND BRAIN DEVELOPMENT

Humans are not unique in having experience-dependent brains, but what sets us apart from other species is how much and which features of our brain depend on experiences to develop. What sets us apart from many animals is actually what we are *missing* when we are born. When a baby turtle hatches from its egg, it is endowed with all the programs and musculoskeletal mechanisms it needs to survive on its own[3] [HALLIWELL2017]. When a human is first born, it is missing various important features and functions [HARVARDDC1]. We build architecture to perform those functions through our experiences.

As we can see from the orphanage scenario, these children were deprived of building important brain architecture, resulting in less gray and white matter density. This was partly due to a lack of enriching environments: they were stuck in cribs and could not navigate other environments or experience various stimuli. However, another deprivation component emerged as one of the key aspects of severe impairments in brain development and behavior: *attachment to a caregiver*. It is not only the physical environment that influences human brain development. In fact, many developmental researchers would assert that the feedback comes from adequate and appropriate *social contact* that plays the biggest role in optimal brain development and adaptive human behavior [SCHORE1994; CACCIOPO2015; FELDMAN2017]. The relational nature of building our brain plays a major role in the unique differences each person has in their response to stimuli, particularly regarding human communication and interaction. As we will see in the following sections and chapters, this is due to its impact on language development and, perhaps more importantly, self-regulatory systems. Impairments to our ability to regulate our affective state are so far-reaching in terms of human behavior and communication that communication cannot be adequately addressed without the topic of self-regulation.

The systems needed to regulate our internal state are not preprogrammed into us. The frontal cortex plays a significant role in these types of systems. These systems are wired and imprinted according to events that happen at the interpersonal and intrapersonal levels. Allan Schore, a leading expert in the field of developmental neuroscience, affirms that systems needed for self-regulation are not accessible at birth and do not emerge spontaneously [SCHORE1994]. They are systems that develop postnatally through social contact [SCHORE1994]. Like many other adaptive human abilities, self-regulation and language are primarily experience-dependent. Like many other adaptive human abilities, self-regulation and language are heavily influenced

---

[3] Interestingly, new research reveals that reptiles that give live birth have higher sociality and the beginnings of what resembles family structures compared with reptiles that lay eggs, Halliwell, B. et al., (2017). "Live bearing promotes the evolution of sociality in reptiles."

by experiences. Because of this, the people in our earliest environments played a significant role in developing our emotion regulation and communication skills.

Off-loading and Outsourcing

Imagine if, just like the baby turtle hatching out of its egg, we came out of the womb with enough "codes" embedded into our neural architecture to help us find our own food, self-regulate, and function completely on our own without a caregiver. This may sound like an ideal situation to some people, but this scenario has trade-offs. An extreme dependency on genes means less flexible "programs" for adapting to changing circumstances [TEGMARK2017; SAPOLSKY2017].

The wait-and-see approach of human development gives us a high level of flexibility to adapt to our specific circumstances. However, it also increases our vulnerability to threats. Without having all of the needed architecture for self-regulation, problem-solving, and communication, a human baby would not survive for long on its own. To deal with this, nature employs the strategy of "outsourcing" or "off-loading." Instead of an infant having all of the needed algorithms already loaded into the genetic code, it can come out of the womb with a template that makes it possible to learn as it goes. This learning mechanism allows a newborn to build models based on imprinting from the people around it. It is also energy-efficient: the imprinting it receives will be based on the movements, strategies, and behaviors the caregivers have been using thus far to survive in that particular environment.

Outsourcing some of our abilities has another benefit. Before leaving the womb, no particular decision-making is required to find sustenance, shelter, or basic life regulation. When you leave this behind, you enter an air-filled space with millions of foreign frequencies and vibrations that hit the sensory receptors in your skin, eyes, nose, mouth, and ears. Your brain can only focus on one thing at a time [DEHAENE2010]. At this point, your brain-body has no reference system yet of what to make of all this data—there is no link between what is worth approaching and what should be avoided for your continued survival. As each second passes, the brain is getting more feedback to help it create associations and algorithms for dealing with all of these stimuli. For example, opening up the airway and letting air pass through the glottis creates a sound (a cry or scream), which is then potentially followed by a sense of pressure and warmth from someone's touch. Shutting the eyelids blocks out light, thus lowering the amount of incoming data. Imagine how much trial and error would be needed to navigate even just a few moments' worth of completely unfamiliar data. Moreover, as infants, our ability to move in this new air-based medium is extremely limited. We must now contend with gravity, inertia, and momentum in order to approach opportunities and avoid threats to our survival. These movement-related mechanisms require bone and muscle development, which take time.

While these are developing, a human infant must have another way to:

1. Protect against threats (external predators, environmental threats, and internal threats from bacteria, infection, and viruses).

2. Ingest necessary nutrients.

3. Continue to build problem-solving skills and algorithms for projecting into the future.

To help with our lack of brain-body maturity, our caregivers become actors on our stage with their mature nervous systems, larger size, and repertoire of problem-solving algorithms. We use them to outsource many aspects of life that are needed for our survival that we do not yet have the neural and behavioral resources to take care of, such as nutrients, shelter, and protection. As our caregivers take care of these for us, our brain-body can ease into its sensory-motor navigation in shorter intervals. This allows our senses to take in vast amounts of unfamiliar data, then withdraw from exteroceptive awareness by sleeping—a process that allows the brain to consolidate information and sensory-motor feedback and procedures [MAQUET2001]. After it has a chance to do this, we can re-enter into exteroceptive awareness and take in more data, then withdraw again from the world to consolidate and integrate. Outsourcing our need for protection from environmental threats allows us to sleep and withdraw awareness to consolidate information. The younger the infant, the more sleep it needs to process the vast amounts of unfamiliar data it is being exposed to.

Serve and Return Feedback

We need to outsource self-protection when we are young and find ways to extract resources and build increasingly complex algorithms and brain circuitry for navigating the world. We do this by creating feedback loops of communication with others to inform them of our needs and internal state. Harvard Center on the Developing Child refers to this as serve and return feedback [HARVARDDC2]. Sending and receiving signals from others is important throughout life. When we are young, this is particularly critical. Because humans lack musculoskeletal mastery for a long time (in contrast to many other species), we are mainly dependent on feedback to survive. Human infants cannot move their body from one location to the next and do not have the muscle strength or control to gather food or move away from danger. To survive during these times of lacking mobility and motor coordination, human children need another human to understand and respond to the signals they are transmitting. This requires four critical features on the part of the caregiver:

1. Mastery of motor coordination and locomotion.

2. An ability to perceive another being's internal state.

3. An understanding of what is needed to alleviate a distressed internal state, extract needed resources, or protect against threat.

4. An understanding that another person has different experiences and resources than the perceiver (e.g., that a newborn does not have teeth and would therefore not be able to chew food). This is called theory of mind, or Social Understanding, which we will examine in Chapter 8.

These four features can only be accumulated with experience and enough data to recognize patterns, which means they require a mature nervous system with a longer history. We cannot meet our needs by pinging out signals to an immature organism that does not have a theory of mind awareness and cannot move its body in ways that can help us navigate challenges and opportunities. If a 6-month-old baby is left in the care of other 6-month-old babies, they will not survive for long. If they do not have the neural and behavioral resources to meet their basic needs, they must find a way to signal for help. This is where communication comes in. The sound of our vocalizations and facial expressions create audible and visible signals for another human to detect what is going on within our internal environment. When a baby cries or screams as they leave the womb, this is the first "ping" out to the world to test this system. It is the first data point that humans create for mastering the various biological tools we have for transmitting signals related to our internal state. If those signals are never "pinged back" or are returned in unpredictable or aversive ways, this creates a lack or gap in data. The development of brain networks tied to the adaptive ability to evaluate changing internal and external environments depends on an infant having enough opportunity for reciprocal social interchanges with a responsive caregiver [SCHORE2003; HARVARDDC2; NSCDC2022].

A lack of or unpredictable "pings" that get returned after we send a signal out means that our brain cannot deduce a clear formula or algorithm that it can rely on to produce a result. If a baby makes a sound and nothing happens, there is a lack of feedback for the brain to adjust its motor commands involved in vocalization, movement, and gesture. To illustrate the importance of the serve-and-return feedback mechanism for developing algorithms and brain circuitry, we can use the example of an infant's first attempts at language.

Let us say you are sitting in your highchair, and you spot a colorful toy on the floor near you. You had already played with this toy and enjoyed its sounds and textures. This created an association of this visual stimulus with a feeling of arousal and stimulation. Because of this, when you see the toy, circuits activate in ways that will drive you to seek that stimulating activity (and the neurochemical state you associate with it) again. But you are unable to reach it or get out of your chair. If there is no one around you in this situation, there may be little you can do to gain access to this toy. This would mean that vocalizing your intention would have no purpose. But since you are a mammal and have experienced human interaction since the moment you were born, you likely have some neural associations with producing sound and observing some feedback in the form of human behavior as a response. If there is a human somewhere in your vicinity, you now have an opportunity to send out a signal and outsource the motor commands of picking up the toy to someone else. At first, however, you do not know which sounds to make to guide their attention to the toy. You have made sounds before, but these sounds generally have elicited attention toward you, not an object. So you make a sound—an attempt to vocalize your desire for the toy (we will discuss gestures and pointing later). Your sound is a signal that becomes part of a feedback loop.

The only way to know which sounds to make will come from trial and error feedback sequences: you ping out a sound, then wait to see what happens. If you make a sound like "ma-ma," you may get back a certain type of movement and vocalization. Depending on how much trial and error you have already engaged in and your motor control over your mouth and tongue, you may try a brand new movement of tongue, lips, glottis, and diaphragm to ping out a sound that sounds like "ba." Suppose this does not elicit a movement from your partner in this situation or a movement unrelated to the toy. In that case, you are gaining feedback that "ma" and "ba" are not the movements you need to make with your tongue, lips, etc., to gain access to the toy. This feedback experience can be made more efficient by two key things: gesture (pointing and/or eye gaze) and modeling. The use of gesture and pointing occurs around 1 year of age. Pointing to the toy and receiving the sound of "toy" from the other person now helps your brain associate a specific sound frequency with the object. You may not have enough motor control to make the full "toy" sound, but if you can get a "t" sound and point, you have a higher chance of guiding the person to give you the toy. The "t" sound has a higher statistical probability of achieving this than the "b" and "m" sound. This gives your brain the data it needs to create statistical inferences, which are sent into its internal working models and algorithms for future behavior.

These sounds and vocal movements get increasingly nuanced as you observe, deduce, and expand your trial-and-error data collection. The people around you also use feedback to understand your sounds. If they reach for a sippy cup when you were trying to indicate the toy, you may start fussing, or turning away. This is data to let them know that they have not "cracked the code" yet of the signals you are emitting. This pinging back and forth of signals is an exchange of data that both parties use to decipher each other's signals.

FEEDBACK AS A TOOL FOR REGULATING NERVOUS SYSTEMS

We see this feedback exchange not only in developing language and problem-solving abilities but also in building self-regulation mechanisms. When the child is born, it uses smell, taste, and touch to interact with its environment. By the end of the second month, occipital areas in the brain become more developed, and there is a dramatic increase in visual perception of human faces [SCHORE1994]. The caregiver's face is one of the most important sources of information for the child. Intense periods of mutual gaze lead the child to track the caregiver in space. This leads the caregiver to look back at the infant, thereby acting as an interpersonal channel for transmitting signals for each person to influence each other [SCHORE1994] mutually. Face-to-face interactions begin at about two months and follow an infant-leads-caregiver sequence [SCHORE1994]. Developmental researchers note that these sequences of face-to-face interactions are highly arousing, full of affective displays that expose infants to vast amounts of social information and dynamic patterns of signals and data [BEEBE1988].

In fact, moment-to-moment analysis of these sequences shows an organized dialog occurring within milliseconds [BEEBE1988]. This dialog means that communication is not only an exchange of information but also a means for the sender to test the responsiveness of the receiver [BRUDZYNSKI2009]. As the infant sends frequencies out to the caregiver and attunes to how these signals are responded to, it gives the infant's brain data on how to make adjustments. The caregivers' responses act as a mirror for the infant's brain to understand itself and what it is doing. Without another face to reflect, the signals would be sent out into the air, and there would be no way for the infant to understand how its micro gestures and movements affect the world around it. This signaling and response is a form of affective synchrony that develops as each partner learns the rhythmic structure and patterns of the other and continuously modifies their behavior to align with those patterns and structures [LESTER1985].

Contingent Responsivity

These feedback loops not only provide information; they also *regulate* the child's physiological arousal. Within face-to-face interactions, the caregiver and child regulate high levels of positive arousal by synchronizing and responding to signals that enhance or dampen the intensity of their affective behavior [FELDMAN1999]. The infant's frontal regions—particularly the orbitofrontal regions—are still in the early stages of their development. Because of this neural "immaturity," the child uses the caregiver's output of facial expressions, voice, and other micromovements as a template for imprinting circuits that form in its own right cortex [SCHORE1994]. This then affects the child's ability to appraise external and internal information [SCHORE1994]. Suppose the caregiver can attend to the infant's cues by adjusting the mode, amount, variability, and timing of stimulation. In that case, this helps the child process changing information according to its actual developmental capacities [SCHORE1994]. In fact, developmental researchers assert that in early infancy, the primary caregiver acts as a child's "auxiliary cortex" [DIAMOND1989]. If there is no mature nervous system capable of adjusting and modulating its signals to enhance or reduce stimulation, the child's brain does not benefit from the experience of emotion regulation and modulation [SCHORE1994; HARVARDDC2]. This is true in situations of neglect or dismissiveness, where the caregiver is unavailable, absent, or inaccessible in some way—whether through altered states due to substances, physical illness, pain, depression, or other mental health challenges [FELDMAN2020].

A lack of modulation and attunement from a caregiver occurs not only in situations of neglect and abuse but also if there is intrusiveness or lack of sensitivity. Studies show that after moments of heightened arousal, the child will avert their gaze to regulate the effects of the intensifying emotion [BEEBE1988].

The caregiver must attune to this and back off to reduce stimulation in these moments. Suppose a caregiver does not tune in to these cues, especially during gaze aversion, and instead continues stimulating the child with their gaze or attention. In that case, this can lead the child to enter a state of distress, which development researcher John Bowlby referred to as protest behavior [FIELD1985]. This misattuned caregiving may lead to a predominance of sympathoexcitatory dopaminergic circuits over the parasympathetic, inhibitory noradrenergic circuits [SCHORE1994]. This type of circuitry dominance may lead to a bias of high-arousal states, avoidance of low-arousal states, and an inefficient capacity to regulate high levels of anger and distress [SCHORE1994]. The more the caregiver tunes their moment-to-moment activity to coordinate with the infant's activity, the more the infant can recover from heightened arousal and learn that it is an effective agent in regulating arousal and stimulation.

LOCOMOTION CHANGES THE COMMUNICATION PATTERNS OF THE CAREGIVER-CHILD RELATIONSHIP

Because we lack musculoskeletal mastery during our first phases of life, proximity to our caregivers remains an essential part of our survival. Face-to-face interaction and eye gaze are major in building the child's emotion regulation neural circuitry. In the latter part of the first year of life, an important event adds another level of complexity to the communication and relational dynamics of the caregiver-child relationship: the infant gains an upright posture and the ability to *locomote independently*. Locomotion allows us to move independently as individuals and gain mastery of new territories that may offer opportunities for beneficial resources. The more expansive the territory, the more options for resources become available. Because a child begins to move further and further away from the physical protection of the caregiver, a new mechanism is now needed for the child to stay safe and capitalize on opportunities within its environment. This new mechanism must be able to travel across air-filled distances. Airborne communication increases the child's chance of survival by allowing it to send and receive signals to and from its caregiver for assessing a potential threat or benefit from something occurring in its environment.

Social Referencing

Moreover, the child is still in the early stages of mastering their musculoskeletal system and gathering data to create algorithms to assess potential threats and opportunities. Therefore, The caregiver must transition out of a role mainly focused on emotional attunement and proximity to a role as a reference point. At 10–12 months, the emergence of social referencing occurs [BRETHERTON1985; WALDEN1988]. Social referencing is a socioemotional function of gaze where the child "reads" the caregiver's face for emotional information about the physical environment [SCAIFE1975]. At this same time, we also see increased joint visual attention[4] when the child first exhibits pointing [BUTTERWORTH1991]. One example of joint attention as a mechanism for social referencing occurs when a child points to an object but checks the other person's gaze [MASUR1983]. This mechanism can be so synchronized that it is called a "shared visual reality" [SCAIFE1975]. It allows the child to see the world from the adult's point of view, which also means that much of what it is experiencing is influenced by how the adult perceives the world. As we will explore throughout this book, our perception of the world is tied to the many social and other factors that have been a part of our experience.

Social referencing means that adult signals heavily influence children's evaluations of the world. Moving away from the caregiver allows the child to explore larger and larger spheres of territory. Communication will enable it to stay safe and continue to benefit from the historical data-based algorithms of its caregiver. In social referencing, the caregiver directly influences the infant's learning of how to feel, how intensely to feel, and whether to feel about objects, people, and environments [WALDEN1988, FEINMAN1982; SCHORE1994]. An example of this can be illustrated in a caregiver-child dyad's first experience with a bumblebee. If this is the first time the child has seen a bee, the novelty of this moving object will likely attract their attention as they observe it move from flower to flower. If the caregiver has had a negative experience with a bee, such as being stung, there is a chance that they will display emotion that conveys a level of fear, avoidance, and/or anxiety. The caregiver may abruptly pick up the child and run away or move the child in a way that indicates a need for protection from the bee. The child has no other template of how to respond to the sight of a bee. The emotional response of the caregiver serves as a template for guiding the child's future responses, which is part of an associative network form of learning that we will explore further in Chapter 8. Suppose the child has multiple other experiences during this time period with other people who are not afraid of bees

---

[4] We will explore joint attention further in Chapter 7.

and who instead sit and observe the bee moving from flower to flower. In that case, the child will have a variety of templates of responses to this stimulus. As generally happens with most children, however, there is not a wide variety of caregivers in the first years of life. So many childhood experiences with various environmental objects and people will be directly influenced by one or two caregivers.

The caregiver's appraisal of objects in the environment influences the development of the internalized system in the infant that assesses the salience and meaning of environmental events and stimuli [SCHORE1994]. These events and the associated signals we observe from those around us create personally meaningful and relevant associations of aspects of the world around us. This leads us to create many shared evaluations of the world with the people who are first in our life, where we look to them to teach and imprint us with what to avoid and approach and how intensely to react to stimuli. This means that many of our appraisals of the world and people around us are not objective; they are imprints of the people we grew up with. Our brain's networks for associations, memory, predictive algorithms, anticipatory adjustments, and emotional relevance are being built through our experiences. The emotions and evaluations of the people around us directly influence these experiences. It is worth reflecting on the idea that the animate and inanimate objects that cause us anxiety, fear, or avoidance are not necessarily things that everyone fears or avoids—our reactions may have been imprinted within us by our caregivers.

This brings us back to the orphans. Without mature nervous systems to attune to, these children would struggle to build the brain circuitry needed to regulate their affective states, enhance positive arousal for exploration, or inhibit over-stimulation. The lack of back-and-forth signaling would result in deficiencies in the neural and behavioral resources needed to modulate and flexibly respond to and appraise ongoing changes in the physical and social environment [HARVARDDC2; NSCDC2022; NELSON2019]. The deficiencies of these circuits were demonstrated not only in the orphan's behavior but in the smaller amounts of gray and white matter mass and density of their brains compared to those of nonneglected children [NELSON2007; NELSON2014].

One of the primary features of a "high-resilient" child and its caregivers is the capacity to transition fluidly from positive affect to negative and back to positive [DEMOS1991]. If a caregiver is absent or unable to modulate and endure both their own negative states and the negative or high-intensity states of their child, this can result in a child's poor adaptability in the face of stress [GAENSBAUER1982; MALATESTA-MAGAI1991]. The most important of those experiences are our social-emotional attunement and attachment interactions with a primary caregiver. The orphans in Romania played a massive role in understanding how critical our first experiences are for building brain circuitry for adapting to challenges. Through many decades of research on emotion regulation, psychopathology, attachment, and developmental neuroscience, we continue to learn that our earliest attachment experiences may be one of the most far-reaching and influential aspects of human behavior across the lifespan.

SUMMARY

Just as we cannot truly understand an organism's evolution and behavior without considering its internal, external, and intertwined biomes, we cannot truly understand human communication without understanding what it is for and what influences it. As we saw from this chapter, the experience-dependent nature of human brain development means that each individual trajectory is influenced by what goes on inside and around us. These trajectories filter into each moment of communication and interact with the build-up of accumulated history and experiences of another person. These experiences affect how we perceive, process, and express what we think, feel, and value. In the next section, we will look at how all of these interacting past experiences may lead to distortions in communication by altering and affecting the signals we transmit and perceive.

REFERENCES

[ACKOFF1978] Ackoff, R. (1978). *The Art of Problem Solving: Accompanied by Ackoff's Fables*. Wiley.

[BAEDKE2020] Baedke, J., Fabregas-Tejeda, A., and Delgado, A. N. (2020). The holobiont concept before Margulis. *Jez-B Molecular and Developmental Evolution: Commentary and Perspective, https://doi.org/10.1002/jez.b.22931*.

[BEEBE1988], Beebe, B., and Lachman, F. M. (1988). The contribution of mother-infant mutual influence to the origins of self- and object relationship. *Progress in Self Psychology*, 3, 3–25.

[BENIGHT2006], Benight, C. C., et al. (2006). Coping self-efficacy as a mediator of distress following a natural disaster. *Journal of Applied Social Psychology* 29(12), 2443–2464.

[BONANNO2013] Bonanno, G. A., and Burton, C. L. (2013). Regulatory flexibility: an individual differences perspective on coping and emotion regulation, *Perspectives on Psychological Science.*

[BRETHERTON1985] Bretherton, I. (1985). Attachment theory: retrospect and prospect. *Monographs of the Society for Research in Child Development*, 50, 3–35.

[BRICKMAN1978] Brickman, P. Coates, D., and Janoff-Bulman, R. (1978). Lottery winners and accident victims: is happiness relative? *Journal of Personality and Social Psychology*, 8, 917–927.

[BRUDZYNSKI2009] Brudsynski, S. (Ed.) (2009). *Handbook of Mammalian Vocalization: An Integrative Neuroscience Approach.* Academic Press.

[BUTTERWORTH1991] Butterworth, G.E. (1991). The ontogeny and phylogeny of joint visual attention. In A. Whiten (Ed.), *Natural theories of mind* (pp. 223–232). Oxford: Basil Blackwell.

[CACIOPPO2015] Cacioppo, J. T., et al. (2015). The neuroendocrinology of social isolation. *Annual Review of Psychology,* 66, 733–767.

[DEHAENE2010] Dehaene, S. (2010). *Consciousness and the brain: deciphering how the brain codes our thoughts.* New York, New York: Viking Press.

[DEMOS1991] Demos, V. (1991) Resiliency in infancy. In T. F. Dugan & R. Coles (Eds.), *The child in our times: Studies in the development of resiliency* (pp. 3–17). New York: Brunner/Mazel.

[DIAMOND1989] Diamond, A., and Doar, B. (1989) The performance of human infants on a measure of frontal cortex function, the delayed response task. *Developmental Psychobiology*, 22, 271–294.

[DOSITS2022] Discovery of Sound in the Sea, University of Rhode Island and Inner Space Center. *https://dosits.org/.*

[ERULKAR2023] Erulkar, Solomon D., and Lentz, Thomas L. (2003) "Nervous system". Encyclopedia Britannica, 22 Jun. 2023, *https://www.britannica.com/science/nervous-system.* Accessed 9 July 2023.

[FEINMAN1982] Feinman, S. (1982). Social referencing in infancy. *Merrill-Palmer Quarterly*, 28, 445–470.

[FELDMAN2020] Abraham, E., Zagoory-Sharon, O., Feldman, R. (2021). Early maternal and paternal caregiving moderates links between preschoolers' reactivity and regulation and maturation of the HPA-immune axis. *Developmental Psychology*, 63, 1482–1498.

[FELDMAN2017] Feldman, R. (2016). The neurobiology of human attachments. *Trends in Cognitive Neuroscience*, (21), 2, *https://doi.org/10.1016/j.tics.2016.11.007*,

[FELDMAN1999] Feldman, R., Greenbaum, C. W., and Yirmiya, N. (1999). Mother-infant affect synchrony as an antecedent of the emergence of self-control. *Developmental Psychology*, 35, 223–231.

[FIELD1985] Field (1985). Attachment as psychobiological attunement: Being on the same wavelength. In M. Reite and T. Field (Eds.), *The psychobiology of attachment and separation* (pp. 415–454). Orlando, FL: Academic Press.

[FOX2010] Fox, S. E., Levitt, P., and Nelson, C. A. (2010). How the timing and quality of early experiences influence the development of brain architecture. *Child Development*, (81). *https://doi.org/10.1111/j.1467-8624.2009.01380.x*.

[GAENSBAUER1982] Gaensbauer, T. J. (1982). Regulation of emotional expression in infants from two contrasting caretaking environments. *Journal of the American Academy of Child Psychiatry*, 21, 163–171.

[GELLHORN1967] Gellhorn, E. (1967). Interruption of behavior, inescapable shock, and experimental neurosis: A neurophysiologic analysis. *Conditional Reflex* 2, 285–293. *https://doi.org/10.1007/BF03034127*.

[HALLIWELL2017] Halliwell, B., et al., (2017). Live bearing promotes the evolution of sociality in reptiles. *Nature Communications* (8), 2030. *https://doi.org/10.1038/s41467-017-02220-w*

[HARREWIJN2021] Harrewijn, A., Abend, R., Naim, R., Haller, S. P., Stavish, C. M., Bajaj, M. A., Matsumoto, C., Dombek, K., Cardinale, E.M., Kircanski, K., and Brotman. M. A. (2021). Attention bias to negative versus non-negative faces is related to negative affectivity in a transdiagnostic youth sample. *Journal of Psychiatric Research*, 138, 514–518.

[HARVARDDC1] Harvard Center on the Developing Child, Experience Builds Brain Architecture: *https://developingchild.harvard.edu/science/key-concepts/brain-architecture/* Accessed 9 July 2023.

[HARVARDDC2] Harvard Center on the Developing Child, Serve and Return Interaction Shapes Brain Circuitry: *https://developingchild.harvard.edu/science/key-concepts/serve-and-return/* Accessed 9 July 2023.

[LANGHE2017] Langhe, B., Puntoni, S., and Larrick, R. (2017). Linear thinking in a non-linear world. *Harvard Business Review https://hbr.org/2017/05/linear-thinking-in-a-nonlinear-world*. Retrieved June 2022.

[HESS1949] Hess, W. (1949). The central control of the activity of internal organs. *Nobel Lecture* December 12, 1949. *https://www.nobelprize.org/prizes/medicine/1949/hess/lecture/*

[KEMPERMANN2019] Kempermann, G. (2019). Environmental enrichment, new neurons and the neurobiology of individuality. *Nature Reviews Neuroscience*, 20, 235–245. *https://doi.org/10.1038/s41583-019-0120-x*

[KOLK22] Kolk, S. M., and Rakic, P. (2022). *Neuropsychopharmacology*, 47, 41–57; *https://doi.org/10.1038/s41386-021-01137-9*

[LESTER1985] Lester, B. M., Hoffman, J., aand Brazleton, T. B. (1985). The rhythmic structure of mother-infant interaction in term and preterm infants. *Child Development*, 56, 15–27.

[MALATESTA-MAGAI1991] Malatesta-Magai, C. (1991) Emotional Socialization: Its role in personality and developmental psychopathology. In D. Cichetti and S. L. Toth (Eds.). *Internalizing and externalizing expressions of dysfunction: Rochester symposium on developmental psychopathology* (pp. 203–224), vol. 2.

[MANDLER1966] Mandler, G., and Watson, D. L. (1966). Anxiety and the interruption of behavior. In: Spielberger, C. D. (Ed.). *Anxiety and behavior* (pp. 263–288). New York, Academic Press.

[MAQUET2001] Maquet, P. (2001). The role of sleep in learning and memory, *Science*, 294, 5544, 1048–1052.

[MASUR1983] Masur, E. F. (1983). Gestural development, dual-directional signaling, and the transition to words. *Psychosomatic Medicine*, 63, 387–401.

[NSCDC2012] National Scientific Council on the Developing Child (2012). *The Science of Neglect: The Persistent Absence of Responsive Care Disrupts the Developing Brain: Working Paper No. 12.* Retrieved from *www.developingchild.harvard.edu*

[NC2022] *https://projects.ncsu.edu/cals/course/ent425/library/tutorials/beha vior/tactile.html*

[NELSON007] Nelson III, C. A., Zeanah, C. H., Fox, N. A., Marshall, P. J., Smyke, A. T., and Guthrie, D. (2007). Cognitive recovery in socially deprived young children: the Bucharest Early Intervention Project. *Science*, 318(5858), 1937–2940.

[NELSON2014] Nelson, C. A., Fox, N. A., and Zeanah, C. H. (2014). *Romania's abandoned children: deprivation, brain development, and the struggle for recovery*. Cambridge, MA, and London, England: Harvard University Press.

[NELSON2019] Nelson, C. A., Zeanah, C. H., and Fox, N. A. (2019). How early experience shapes human development: the case of psychosocial deprivation. *Hindawi Neural Plasticity https://doi.org/10.1155/2019/1676285*.

[PAYNE2015] Payne P., and Crane-Godreau, M. A. (2015). The preparatory set: a novel approach to understanding stress, trauma, and the bodymind therapies.. *Frontiers in Neuroscience*

[RAFFERTY2023] Rafferty, John P. (2023). Thorndike's law of effect. *Encyclopedia Britannica, 7 April 2023, https://www.britannica.com/science/ Thorndikes-law-of-effect*. Accessed 9 July 2023.

[SAPOLSKY2017] Sapolksy, R. (2017) *Behave: the biology of humans at their best and worst*. New York, NY: Penguin Press.

[SCAIFE1975], Scaife, M. & Brunder, J. S. (1975). The capacity for joint visual attention in the infant. *Nature*, 253, 265–266.

[SCHORE1994] Schore, A. (1994) *Affect regulation and the origin of the self: the neurobiology of emotional development*. Hillsdale, NJ: Erlbaum.

[SHOOK2007] Shook, N. J., Fazio, R. H., and Vasey, M. W. (2007). Negativity bias in attitude learning: A possible indicator of vulnerability to emotional disorders? *Journal of Behavior Therapy and Experimental Psychiatry*, 38(2), 144–155.

[STROEBE2010] Stroebe, M., and Schut, H. (2022). The dual process model of coping with bereavement: a decade on. *Omega (Westport)*, 61(4), 273–289. *https://doi.org/10.2190/OM.61.4.b*. PMID: 21058610.

[TEGMARK2017] Tegmark, M. (2017) *Life 3.0: Being Human in the Age of Artificial Intelligence*. Penguin Books Limited.

[VANDERWERT2010] Vanderwert, R. E., et al., (2010). Timing of intervention affects brain electrical activity in children exposed to severe psychosocial neglect. *PLoS One. https://doi.org/10.1371/journal.pone.0011415*

[WALDEN1988] Walden, T. A., and Ogan, T. A. (1988). The development of social referencing. *Child Development*, 59, 1230–1240.

[WOODWORTH1918] Woodworth, R. S. (1918). *Dynamic psychology*. New York: Columbia University Press.

[ZUG2022] Zug, George R. (2003). Locomotion. *Encyclopedia Britannica*, 30 July 2022, *https://www.britannica.com/topic/locomotion*. Accessed 9 July 2023.

CHAPTER

2

SIGNAL DISTORTION: UNCONSCIOUS FILTERS THAT BIAS COMMUNICATION AND PERCEPTION

When we think of someone overreacting, what do we mean by this exactly? If we notice someone yelling, pointing, withdrawing, or not responding to our efforts to communicate, how does this affect our subsequent decision in that interaction? So much of what happens in our social exchanges is tied to how we perceive what is happening before us. Are those perceptions truly accurate? Are we seeing and hearing things around us as they really are? Or are other forces at play? In the previous chapter, we saw how early experiences can influence our abilities to dampen or excite our states of arousal. We also saw how our early forms of detecting signals from caregivers play a role in how we evaluate and judge the world around us. In this chapter and future chapters, we will see that our ability to regulate our responses to events and stimuli flexibly greatly impacts the frequencies and signals we transmit, detect, and interpret during communicative interactions with others. Nervous system regulation is, therefore, an inseparable part of communication.

Regulating our responses is tied heavily to our ability to detect threats and opportunities appropriately. Because of the many experience-dependent and unconscious forces playing a role in our perceptions and interpretations, we may interpret events as more threatening than they actually are. In some cases, we may also underestimate the harm a situation or person may cause us. Using too much or insufficient energy for defense and protection than is necessary is a form of maladaptive response. On the other hand, adaptive coping mechanisms occur when there is a match between our energy expenditure and situational requirements. This means that when something is not life-threatening, we are not expending energy and resources as though it is. It means we are not "over-reacting." On the flip side, it also means that we are not "under-reacting," meaning that when life presents challenges and opportunities, we do not under-expend energy and resources to benefit from or navigate them.

Energy expenditure can relate to the intensity and/or duration of a response. An example of this would be someone stubbing their toe on a coffee table and staying emotionally dysregulated after the physical pain has subsided. In this scenario, the potential threat is the injury of the toe. If that has been resolved and the person is still distressed, the energy allocated to their distressed state is not accessible for other actions and problem-solving. Without realizing it on a conscious level, a person may feel upset about stubbing their toe because of various associations being made with the event. Perhaps they did not see the coffee table because they were preoccupied with other thoughts, and these preoccupations were due to feeling overwhelmed and anxious. From there, various associated thoughts may turn to thoughts of blame or being overwhelmed that their partner or family members are not supporting them in ways they would find helpful. Or it may turn to an internalization of responsibility; the person becomes angry at themselves for being disorganized, unable to deal with stress, etc. The emotion regulation and attachment theory field reveals that many of our current struggles related to dysregulated states and disproportionate reactions to events often have roots associated with our past [SCHORE1994]. Events in our present experiences can also trigger implicit processes related to misattuned social experiences in our history and may trigger intense arousal dysregulation [SCHORE1994]. Severe dysregulation occurring in response to events that are not life-threatening may be an inefficient allocation of energy and resources, which reflects challenges in a mechanism known as regulatory flexibility [BONNANO2013].

REGULATORY FLEXIBILITY

Dysregulated and disproportionate responses are an indication of challenges in response flexibility. Due to the constantly shifting demands of our environment and the complexity and unpredictability of human-to-human interaction, the ability to *shift* strategies according to emerging challenges and opportunities is one of the keys to our survival and thriving. Rather than

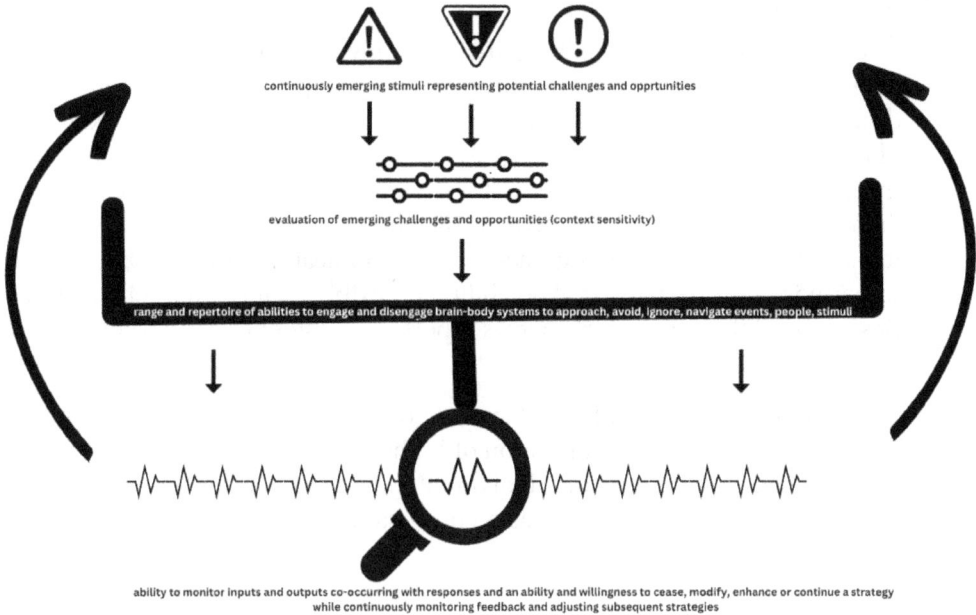

continuously emerging stimuli representing potential challenges and opprtunities

evaluation of emerging challenges and opportunities (context sensitivity)

range and repertoire of abilities to engage and disengage brain-body systems to approach, avoid, ignore, navigate events, people, stimuli

ability to monitor inputs and outputs co-occurring with responses and an ability and willingness to cease, modify, enhance or continue a strategy while continuously monitoring feedback and adjusting subsequent strategies

adopting a uniform strategy to navigate challenges, adopting *flexibility itself* as a strategy is a crucial component for health, well-being, and adjustment [BONANNO2013]. Flexibility is what makes a system robust. It is a continuously changing, responsive, and multifaceted adjustment to stressor variability [BONANNO2013]. The idea of flexibility contrasts what Bonanno and colleagues propose as the "fallacy of uniform efficacy." This fallacy points to a misguided idea that one strategy experienced as effective in one context would make it automatically effective in all contexts. The concept of regulatory flexibility, on the other hand, describes the ability to perceive subtle contextual shifts and new demands and opportunities and then to shift and explore appropriate strategies to regulate our systems in the face of those demands and opportunities [BONANNO2013]. Adaptive social behavior and communication patterns help individuals flexibly transition between states and energy expenditures. In contrast, a lack of variability in response to changing conditions would be a feature of pathological or maladaptive behavior [SCHORE1994].

Regulatory flexibility includes three main components: context sensitivity, a repertoire of strategies, and an ability to monitor and respond to feedback [BONNANO2013].

Context Sensitivity

The first step in flexible self-regulation involves evaluating emerging challenges and opportunities. A sensitive and accurate perception of nuances and differences or similarities within each new situation increases the likelihood of choosing an appropriate strategy to deal with it. Lack of context sensitivity means that a person may perceive, for example, a social interaction as threatening when the context is not actually dangerous. On the other hand, perceiving a situation as safe when in fact there are indicators of impending danger or harm is also problematic. The ability to flexibly nuance and detect subtleties within different contexts allows a person to use energy more efficiently. Examples of this include the ability to:

- Respond with sympathoexcitatory activity when a situation is life-threatening and requires mobilization of limbs;
- Detect that a situation may feel threatening due to social factors but is not physically dangerous, such as a conversation where there is a perceived rejection;
- Move from a sense of safety and parasympathetic dominance to alertness and sympathetic system activation when appropriate—such as being on a date, party, or public setting and noticing that another person's signals may indicate boundary violation or potentially harmful behavior.

In those contexts, the flexibility to suppress or enhance sympathoexcitatory activity is needed to respond appropriately. Context sensitivity allows a person to evaluate a given situation so that their choice of response strategy matches the level of challenge or opportunity presented at each moment.

Context Insensitivity

Emotion context insensitivity has been linked with a variety of mental health challenges such as anxiety and depression [COIFMAN2010; GEHRICKE2000; LARSON2007; ROTTENBERG2007; 2004; 2005]. In studies on depression that explore context sensitivity, the inability to modulate sadness and grief according to contexts is associated with poorer functioning and higher levels of depressive symptoms. In one study, for example, participants who were depressed reported the same feelings of sadness after watching a sad film as the nondepressed patients but felt more sorrow than nondepressed participants after watching a neutral movie [ROTTENBERG2002]. It was not their baseline sadness that explained their poorer functioning, but their inability to modulate it according to different contexts [ROTTENBERG2002]. The failure to modulate sadness may mean that a person is continuing to perceive a situation in a way that has a strong negative bias. In doing so, they may miss opportunities to engage in flexible cognitive processes for seeing current sources of optimism, support, and pathways forward.

Context insensitivity can also damage relationships, such as when a person expresses anger in a situation that requires rapport-building or repair [BONANNOKELTNER1997; COLE1992; KELTNER1993]. Maladaptive or dysfunctional emotional responses are a mismatch, insufficient, or go beyond the actual demands of the situation [GOLDSMITH2004]. The better we perceive nuances in context, the more choices we have to respond flexibly. For example, an interaction may be uncomfortable—such as receiving a critique—but that is different than receiving a threat of physical harm or even rejection (a friend or partner critiquing does not necessarily mean they are trying to end the relationship). Suppose a person is not sensitive to the nuances of these contexts and perceives them all as equally threatening. In that case, they will have less variability in their strategies for responding and have a higher likelihood of responding maladaptively, such as ending a relationship or abandoning a project after receiving a critique. Context sensitivity is only one aspect of a flexible response, however. To expend energy appropriately and efficiently, a person must also have the capacity to enact a variety of strategies. This ability is tied to the concepts of range and repertoire.

Repertoire

The strategies a person has at their disposal during a given situation constitutes their repertoire. There are three key aspects to the robustness of a repertoire: size, temporal variability, and type. Size relates to the number of strategies. Studies reveal that a higher number is linked with resilient trajectories [BONNANO2013]. Temporal variability is related to using coping strategy at different time points, such as in preparation for, during, and after an interaction or event. Categorical variability includes the ability to shift from enhancing or suppressing emotions, focusing on the emotions, or solving the problem causing the emotions [FOLKMAN2000; LAZARUS1984]. One area of research on this is in the dual process model of grief, where the ability to navigate the loss of a loved one is related to engagement strategies, such as using photos or music as reminders of the person, as well as disengagement strategies such as plans for life without them and connecting with people not associated with that person [STROEBE2010].

Feedback

Another critical element to flexible responding and system regulation is feedback. Within a system, feedback is needed to monitor and modify whether a strategy needs to be adjusted, maintained, or ceased. As an illustration, let us look at a thermostat-heater system. The purpose of this system is to keep a room at a temperature determined by entering a number into the thermostat. The furnace will turn on (initiate) or turn off (inhibit) at various intervals to keep the room's temperature at the desired level. The furnace cannot function on its own. Without feedback about the temperature in the room, it does not have the information needed to determine if it should turn on or off. Feedback is necessary for it to be regulated.

Even the most robust repertoire of strategies is not enough to create maximum flexibility and systems resilience if there is no way to monitor whether a plan is effective [BONANNO2001; SCHERER2009; SHEPPES2012]. Monitoring how communication is received is crucial for knowing whether one should maintain the current strategy or readjust. For example, if you are speaking with someone, their responses to you allow you to adjust or maintain the current strategy you are using to communicate. If you are joking, and they nod, smile, and respond in words that match the context, you have feedback that can allow you to stay on course. If you are sharing something that distresses or saddens you and you would like to be comforted—but instead, they laugh, this also gives feedback that the current communication strategy is not creating the desired response. To meet your goal of finding comfort and reassurance, your subsequent strategy may be to end the conversation and find a different person to speak with or adjust how you are expressing or managing your sadness. Your repertoire gives you access to multiple options for responding according to the feedback you are receiving. Three particular aspects of feedback are important to our understanding of self-regulation and its role in communication dynamics: internal feedback, social feedback, and feedback responsiveness.

Internal Feedback

One type of internal feedback occurs within various systems of the brain and body. Information from our senses, viscera, peripheral and central nervous system is communicated within feedback loops so the brain can use inhibition to sculpt neural activity in ways appropriate for the context [KNIGHT1999; THAYER2005]. This is also known as interoception [CAMERON2001].

According to Thayer and Lane, the conscious experience of emotion involves signal transmission from subcortical areas to the cerebral cortex, as well as top-down inhibitory influences from the cerebral cortex to the subcortical centers [THAYER2009]. Without these internal feedback systems, the brain-body does not receive bottom-up information from the senses and cannot issue top-down commands to our autonomic and somatic nervous systems to contract, expand, inhibit, or initiate movements within our organs and skeletal muscles to help us navigate each situation.

Internal feedback allows us to monitor our own regulation strategies in the face of stressors. It allows us to *feel* whether our actions and expressions are creating a desired internal state. An example of this would be if someone had a fear of public speaking and decided to face their fear by giving a speech at a dinner party. As they are about to give the speech, they feel their face flush, their throat getting dry, and their palms sweating. They feel their vocal muscles tighten and constrict, and they have difficulty breathing. The awareness of these sensations is due to communication between various internal systems such as the viscera and the central nervous system. If this person has a repertoire of strategies, they may choose in that moment to use one of them, such as cognitive reappraisal (telling themselves there is nothing to fear; it is all in their mind) or perhaps mindful noticing (focusing on the feelings of the heart beating fast and the face flushing). If they try one of these strategies and still feel like their throat is cramping and they cannot speak, this feedback is what tells them to cease or modify their current strategy and implement a new one. If they have a repertoire of engagement and disengagement, they may then try to distract themselves by looking at the light of a candle nearby, at a small child sitting at the table, or at the back of the wall above everyone's faces. If this strategy leads to a slower heart beat, relaxing of their muscle tension, and an ability to speak calmly, they can maintain this strategy, and this feedback can be used to continue the use of the strategy. Some research indicates that in high-intensity emotional situations, people tend to prefer distraction or disengagement over engagement strategies [SHEPPES2012]. If someone is afraid of flying and encounters turbulence and their distress levels become extremely high, for example, they may choose to distract themselves first with stimuli that move them away from noticing the turbulence, and then as their distress level lowers, they may be better able to engage in cognitive reappraisals or mindful breathing [SHEPPES2012]. Their internal feedback is what allows them to know at each moment if a strategy is working to regulate their state into a desired level of arousal. This desired level is relative: if a person is overwhelmed, they may desire to feel calmer. If their internal state is dissociated or disengaged, lethargic, frozen, they may have a desire to increase arousal in their internal environment in order to take action. A key insight from regulatory flexibility research is that a range of engagement and disengagement, inhibition, and arousal strategies can be useful for regulating the nervous system.

Social Feedback

As we saw in the previous chapter, feedback from the social milieu is a crucial source of self-regulation [COLE1994]; [EISENBERG1992]; [RYAN1997]. When one animal or person sends out signals, it is the responses and behavioral consequences of the receiver that gives the sender clues as to the effectiveness of its communicatory process [BRUDZYNSKI2010]. Multiple feedback loops are involved in communication: the sender's expressions influence and incite responses from the receiver, and these responses then influence the behavior of the sender [COTE2005].

Feedback Responsiveness

As we monitor and receive constantly changing feedback, we also need to flexibly integrate the information into our subsequent behaviors. This flexibility is tied to *feedback responsiveness* [KATO2012]. It includes the ability to flexibly assess, re-assess situational demands and opportunities, continue effective strategies, and discontinue ineffective strategies or implement alternatives on an ongoing basis. Research on feedback responsiveness highlights two major dimensions [KATO2012]:

Evaluation—the sensitivity to the efficacy of a strategy (e.g., being aware of how successful or unsuccessful one's attempts to communicate have been).

Adaptiveness—the willingness to implement other strategies (e.g., if a stressful situation has not improved, a person tries to think of other ways to cope with it).

Research has shown feedback responsiveness as being predictive of flexible thinking and positive mental health outcomes [KATO2012].

The key to a resilient and optimally performing system is its ability to match energy expenditure to situational requirements (context sensitivity). In order to do this, a system must have a repertoire of strategies to draw from that may engage or inhibit various mechanisms for appropriate energy expenditure (repertoire). This is a dynamic and ongoing process that also requires the system to know when its strategies are having the desired result or not. Feedback is a crucial component of this entire system. Feedback is internally based, such as the visceral sensations we get as we think about things, and externally based, as our senses interact with external stimuli such as the movements, gestures, and signals being transmitted by the people around us (social feedback). These feedback loops build the regulatory features of our brain-body system. As we will see in the next section, however, within this feedback-dependent process, we run into many of our challenges in human communication.

CHALLENGES TO REGULATORY FLEXIBILITY

Due to the relational experience-dependent aspects of our brain and nervous system, several mechanisms within our brain-body systems may hamper our ability to respond adaptively in social interactions. These mechanisms may lead us to lack context sensitivity, such as when we unconsciously perceive an interaction as more threatening than it is. Because of this, we may select a response that does not fit the situation, and we may also narrow our range of what we pay attention to in terms of feedback. This context insensitivity can create a repetitive pattern of maladaptive behavior within relationships and social situations. We may think we are responding to others' signals in ways that are accurate and complete pictures of what is going on; however, many systems are unconsciously directing us to pay attention and make meaning of what we perceive based on our past rather than what is currently occurring.

As we saw in the previous chapter, we are not born with self-regulatory features for coping with stressful situations. The signals being sent back and forth between child and caregiver provide feedback loops that are necessary for the brain to develop architecture related to the inhibitory and other executive functioning mechanisms needed to adjust, monitor, and down-regulate intense emotions so that we engage in exploration and play. We also saw that due to the limited number of people who interact with us during our first experiences, there are limited and often repetitive feedback loops that create limited algorithms and working models that guide our current reactions based on our past experiences.

The social and emotional experiences and communications we have had over the course of our life are a combination of internal state shifts and sequences of movements. Our eyes shifted to meet our caregivers. Their eyes moved to meet ours, or they moved in a different direction. The muscles around their eyes, in their jaw, pharynx and larynx, head and limbs moved in ways that expressed their internal state in response to what they were perceiving with their senses. This sequence of movements led to a certain combination of neurochemical patterns in each person involved in the interaction, perhaps including oxytocin and endogenous feel-good opiates, or perhaps combinations of cortisol and norepinephrine or epinephrine, creating a sense of agitation and distress. If we are around the same people repeatedly for our first years of life, many of these patterns of micro-movements can become a part of a familiar sequence. Sequences of movements can become ingrained into subconscious systems. This learning process leads us to engage in familiar sequences quickly and without a lot of effort or awareness. This concept is related to *procedural memory,* which is a type of memory that stores action patterns associated with different situations and activities.

Implicit and procedural memory

Remember when you first learned to drive a car or ride your bike? In the very first moments of learning how to do these things, you likely would not have been able to focus on other things, such as carrying on a full conversation. As you mastered the sequence of movements and the range of dynamic responses needed to drive or ride your bike, it likely felt like less effort to concentrate on the exact moves you needed to make. As you needed to focus less of your conscious and effortful attention on how to drive or ride, this freed up space for you to attend to other things. Compare how much more comfortable you likely feel about being able to look around or even talk to someone while driving or riding a bike now. After enough practice and repetition, your brain-body found a way to store and retrieve that information in a way that became experientially different than when you first started. This is what learning does for us. With enough exposure and practice, networks and communication patterns within our brain-body system become more automated, which frees up our attention to deal with other things, while our body seems to "take over" [SAPOLSKY2017]. If we had no way of automating the mechanisms for learning, we would constantly need to re-learn and use attentional effort to remember how to do each action in a sequence. Learning requires a lot of focus and attention. When these resources are being used, it is difficult to focus on other things at the same time. As an adaptive system, the brain-body creates automated processes to help free up attentional resources for other goals and behaviors. These unconscious processes can be called "implicit," meaning that they are not something we can access and retrieve consciously or at will.

Implicit memory is in contrast to explicit memory. Explicit memory can be accessed at will. It is something we can be fully conscious of, consider and re-evaluate [PAYNE2015]. It is also known as "declarative memory" and includes memories about personal experiences and factual information [DEW2011]. For example, you can choose to retrieve a memory about what you had for dinner yesterday, the last social gathering you attended, or a vacation you took last year. It may not have all of the details, but you are able to choose to activate the memory to a certain degree.

Examples of explicit or declarative memory are:

- Information about the world and the meaning of words. This is known as semantic memory, e.g., remembering that Lisbon is the capital of Portugal.

- Episodic memory: We can recall details about events we have experienced.

- Spatial memory: Stored information about spatial arrangements, which you can retrieve when needed to find your way in familiar places.

Implicit memory, on the other hand, generally cannot be retrieved in a way that brings it into full conscious awareness. A particular type of implicit memory is procedural memory, which helps us perform tasks by making motor action patterns "second nature" [WILLINGHAM1989].

The Orbital Prefrontal Cortex and Procedural Memory

Research indicates that the orbital prefrontal system plays a major role in procedural memory as well as self-regulatory and socio-affective processes. This system is located at a convergence zone of the cortex and subcortex, giving it access to "virtually any activity taking place in our beings' mind or body at any given moment" [DAMASIO1994, p.181]. This system relates to positive affective states and generates approach behavior via excitatory circuits of the sympathetic nervous system [NAUTA1982]. It is also associated with avoidant behaviors and negative affective states via parasympathetic circuits [SCHORE1994].

This orbitofrontal system also:

- Processes visual and auditory signals, particularly from emotional faces, and integrates these with internal, visceral signals related to emotions and motivations [PANDYA1985].

- Selectively attends to specific aspects of facial expressions [ETCOFF1984].

- Assesses and evaluates facial expressions [AHERN 1991].

- Generates autonomic activity in response to unconsciously perceived facial expressions [JOHNSON1991].

This system for integrating external and internal signals plays a significant role in procedural memory. The types of social–emotional interactions we have when we are young become embodied algorithms that are stored as implicit-procedural memory that relate to how certain situations have been frequently paired with certain emotional responses within each individual's experience [DAMASIO1995]. These past-based algorithms activate procedural processes of approach or avoid mechanisms that may also include an evaluation of a person's ability to cope with what they are perceiving [SCHORE1994].

Past experiences can create emotional associations with sequences of actions we have observed in others. For example, a young child sees their caregiver come home, get something out of the fridge, and then go into a room and close the door. If the child had wanted to interact with that parent and decided to open the living room door but was met with hostility or dismissiveness, this would begin to form a set of data points and associated internal state fluctuations. Because it occurred once, the sequence of fridge-living room-closed door rejection would now be considered as a possible prediction for future interactions. If the child attempted to do this again and were met with the same reaction, this would reinforce that statistical probability even more that this would happen again. If the child opened the door and there was a different response, the possibility would change, and there would be less certainty. Suppose the first encounter with this sequence of events (fridge-living room-closed door rejection) caused distress. In that case, there is also a chance that the child would not attempt to open the door and interact with the parent, resulting in a high statistical probability of rejection (there is no data to contradict it).

This has profound implications for our future responses and approaches to communication and relationship behaviors. A closed door is not a threatening stimulus. But if the experience of this is paired with a fear of misattunement or rejection, a closed door and the sequence of associated behaviors may get stored as a long-term implicit memory, which will activate a state of dysregulation for that person without them knowing why. Moreover, due to a lack of mature circuitry, which would include perspective-taking, a child may deduce a simple cause-effect model that *they* are the cause of the closed door or hostility rather than understanding that the parent has their own stressors unrelated to the child. Their response to a closed door or various action patterns related to this scenario may trigger a sense of rejection. Implicit memories like these regularly "influence behavior without one being conscious of the influence" [ROEDIGER1990]. The orbitofrontal systems play a role in implicit memory as well as enhancing sensitivities to instruct our brain-body system on how to act and what to do in social situations [SCHORE1994]. Because of the experience-dependent nature of this system, what we see, say, and do in social interactions is highly connected to our past [DEECKE1985; PRIBRAM1991].

Anticipation and Preparation

Implicit and procedural memory processes also play a significant role in how we anticipate and prepare for an interaction [PAYNE2015]. Muscle tone, visceral state, and expectations form rapidly and unconsciously through processes that involve our previous experiences. This leads people, as mentioned earlier, to react and decide "emotionally," often based on implicit learning [HOVDESTAD1996; LUETHI2008; ORANGE2011]. This rapid initial appraisal involves implicit and procedural memory to generate a set of expectations about a situation [PAYNE2015]. This is similar to Stephen Porges' concept of neuroception, which he describes as a subcortically, mainly unconscious evaluation of safety or lack of safety in a given situation [PORGES2004].

FEEDBACK, STRESS REGULATION, AND AUTONOMIC RESPONSES

As we communicate and interact with others, these implicit processes influence our internal and social feedback inputs and outputs, such as visceral sensations, eye gaze and direction, facial expressions, posture, and other cues from our face and body. These unconscious appraisals and feedback loops lead to a variety of autonomic nervous system states [LEVINE1977; BERNTSON1994]. The polyvagal theory, proposed by Stephen Porges, suggests the following combinations of autonomic responses in response to unconscious detection and appraisals of social, internal, and environmental cues [PORGES2004]:

▪ Immobility without fear
▪ Immobility with fear

- Fight-or-flight mobilization
- Play
- Social engagement

The above list highlights two basic distinctions of nervous system responses: ergotropic and trophotropic.

Ergotropic generally refers to a response to a challenge. In addition to responding to actual threats, perceiving a situation as challenging can also lead to ergotropic activity. Ergotropic is a term first used by Swiss physiologist W. R. Hess to describe the status of the nervous system that favors energy expenditure [HESS1949]. The simplest example of this is a rapid increase in sympathetic activity that allows for a fight-or-flight response. This ergotropic system activates motor, premotor, endocrine, and central nervous system responses in preparation for strong energy expenditure, which includes [PAYNE2015]:

- Muscle tension prepares the body for action.

- Secretions of stress hormones.

- Heightened sensory awareness.

Trophotropic refers to the status of the nervous system that facilitates rest and restoration of energy stores. An example of this is the parasympathetic "rebound" that occurs following sympathetic (ergotropic) arousal in response to challenge [GELLHORN1970]. In healthy systems, ergotropic activity is followed by restorative trophotropic states. This ergotropic and trophotropic challenge-repair sequence can occur in sudden threatening situations, as well as in sports, vigorous play, and other voluntary recreational activities with an element of risk [EVERLY2013]. In these situations, the ergotropic system has a short-term activation, followed by trophotropic recuperation and rest [GELLHORN1970]. This short-term activation has been referred to as "good" stress [EVERLY2013]. An exposure to stress that is successfully resolved plays a role in stress inoculation [MEICHENBAUM1985] and resilience [KARATSOREOS2013; WU2013]. If our body prepares for stress, it will only result in increased resilience IF it is well-matched to the situation, and the situation can be resolved quickly. [PAYNE2015]. Examples of this could include emergency first responders who receive adequate training and are well prepared for a stressful event and athletes who encounter high activation of sympathetic arousal during a sport. This type of resilience-building ergotropic-trophotropic balance would also play a part in people who encounter stressful social situations, such as at work or at home, as long as those situations are resolved successfully and quickly, and the preparatory response is well-matched to the case; the person is not preparing for a life-threat when the case is not calling for it (context-sensitive).

Under normal conditions, these two systems—sympathetic (ergotropic) and parasympathetic (trophotropic)—interact in reciprocal ways and return to baseline after a challenge [GELLHORN1956]. However, even after moderately intense disturbances, they can become chronically biased to default into a sympathetic or parasympathetic state and have difficulties returning to baseline levels of regulation [PAYNE2015A], a mechanism called "tuning" [GELLHORN1967]. Gellhorn's seminal work on nervous system responses in animals revealed that when rats underwent stress below a certain threshold, they displayed a temporary increase in sympathetic activity (with lower parasympathetic activation) and then returned to baseline levels. However, if the stressor exceeded a certain threshold in intensity and duration, the rats' autonomic nervous system did not return to baseline. Instead, the rats remained in a chronic, elevated sympathetic (ergotropic) state [GELLHORN1967].

If stressful conditions last longer, are more chronic, or are more intense than an organism's neural and behavioral capacity to tolerate it, the system can become "biased" or "tuned" in one direction [GELLHORN1967]. This diminishes its capacity to respond flexibly to future events using a repertoire of engagement or disengagement strategies. These deleterious neurochemical effects refer to allostatic load [LUPIEN2006]. Allostatic load relates to the cost or wear and tear of chronic, persistent exposure to heightened endocrine responses that result from needing to continuously adapt to repeated challenges that the individual experiences as stressful [MCEWEN2007, MCEWEN2010].

The challenge with a developing brain and nervous system in a young human is that if stressors occur within its first environment, there is a good chance that the child will be chronically exposed to those stressors over a relatively long period. In contrast to many other species, the period of dependency on a caregiver is extremely long for humans. Much of that is due to the complexity and adaptability of the human prefrontal cortex, which requires many years to develop [SAPOLSKY2017]. As we saw in the previous chapter, this long developmental period of critical brain-body networks means that human children need to outsource much of their regulation abilities to their caregivers. A human child does not have the neural and behavioral systems to function independently outside of the situation they find themselves in. Since we do not come equipped with automated mechanisms, and we have a long biological dependency period, if we are in environments with a lack of sensitive and responsive caregiving that enables us to go through challenge-repair/restore sequences, that can lead to challenges and biases in nervous system functioning and a person's later social–emotional functioning. Two environmental factors make humans particularly vulnerable to these challenges: inescapability and repetitive exposure.

Inescapability

An adult has access to multiple options for leaving an undesired situation and finding other sources of co-regulation; a young child does not. A 3-year-old being abused or rejected by a caregiver cannot walk out the door and navigate a different relationship to help them regulate. This means that the interactions occurring within the home represent interactions that are much more threatening to a child's nervous system than to an adult with more sophisticated mobilization and fight-flight mechanisms, as well as more options for relationships to meet their needs. The primary caregiver(s) are all the child has to regulate and build the brain architecture for their own future self-regulation. Rejection and misattunement from a caregiver represent a serious impairment to a child's overall ability to restore their nervous system through the biologically imperative process of co-regulation. Therefore, rejection, abuse, dismissiveness, and hostility represent a "life threat" to the child. A child's overall functioning and ability to survive and thrive are in danger without access to a caregiver who can attune to its needs. A child cannot leave a home environment, even if it is stressful beyond their capacity to cope. When stress is extreme and *inescapable*, the autonomic nervous system may even undergo extreme activation of the sympathetic and parasympathetic branches at the same time [GELLHORN1964A]. This is believed to be a mechanism underlying tonic immobility, a "deer in headlights" type of response that occurs in both humans and animals where there is co activation of parasympathetic and sympathetic systems with a loss of coping mechanisms [PATON2006; NIJENHUIS1998A; MARX2008]. Tonic immobility can occur when a stressor occurs, but the organism is restrained from escaping or moving and can result in posttraumatic stress symptoms in both humans and animals [BERNSTON1994; MANDLER1966; BOVIN2008]. As mentioned earlier in this chapter, being exposed to levels of stress beyond one's ability to regulate is also related to allostatic load and wear and tear on the nervous system to degrees that can make it increasingly more difficult to rebound after a stressor [LUPIEN2006].

The component of inescapability emerges as a powerful influence on both animal and human stress responses. Rats subjected to stressful stimuli but restrained from escaping have been shown to develop behavioral problems [GELLHORN1967; MANDLER1966]. In studies by Ledoux and colleagues, if the rats are later placed in the original situation but given a chance to escape from the stressor, the conditioned fear rapidly disappears [LEDOUX2001]. In human experiments, participants instructed not to move when subjected to the startling sound of a pistol shot to stay in an elevated sympathetic state; however, if they are invited to move vigorously, their nervous system rapidly returns to baseline [FREEMAN1942]. Other studies indicate a relationship between inescapable stress and impairments to social responses due to impacts on social reward functions [DANIELS2021]. In human environments, inescapable stress may not be as extreme or controlled as is possible in animal studies. However, these experiments point to how a limitation in being able to use various strategies to withdraw ourselves from a stressful situation can have deleterious neuro-endocrine and behavioral effects.

Repetitive Exposure

Because of the long period of dependency in humans, a child is exposed repetitively and for a long time to a caregiver's patterns of behaviors, internal states, and responses to events. If a caregiver is skilled in self-regulation and attuning to others, this will help the child internalize adaptive strategies for their own self-regulation and future affiliative behavior. If the caregiver lacks context sensitivity, range and repertoire, and feedback responsiveness, however, the child will be exposed to these misattuned behaviors for many years and on a regular basis. This repeated exposure to a misattuned caregiver influences the internal working models that affect how they predict and perceive the world around them.

Predictive Biases

One way this occurs is in how unconscious processes affect our attention. We do not pay conscious attention to all of the inputs that exist around us. To be more efficient, unconscious parallel processes determine which objects are relevant and should be attended to. Various studies have shown that unconscious processes are constantly monitoring what is going on around us and assigning a value that guides what we pay attention to. For example, the brain uses various mechanisms to "tag" what is most relevant to us according to our goals, which then draws our attention [DEHAENE2014]. These attentional biases are tied to implicit, subcortical processes and predictive models. In people who report higher trait anxiety, studies show basolateral amygdala hyperactivity in response to subliminal fearful faces [ETKIN2004]. Suppose a person has a history of unpredictable patterns of attunement and safety or dominance of threat and rejection with a caregiver or family member. In that case, this can affect their expectations and detection of threatening stimuli. For example, veterans' prior exposure to extreme pain has been shown to alter neural responses that make neutral stimuli seem potentially threatening [EIDELMAN2016].

Moreover, negative information is generally given priority over positive information [CACIOPPO1999]. As a default response to uncertainty, novelty, and threat, the brain (and in particular, the amygdala) recruits various systems to serve a vigilance function for biologically relevant information (which can include animals, faces)—both positive and negative—but with a bias toward negative information [CUNNINGHAM2008]. This makes sense from an evolutionary perspective for maximizing survival and adaptive responses: when in doubt, err on the side of caution [LEDOUX1996]. We may lose out on an opportunity, but if we are right about something being a threat, at least we have avoided harm.

This bias toward detecting threats can create challenges within interpersonal communication and interactions. First, these systems are activated in response to uncertainty, novelty, and threat. If we are engaging in a social interaction with someone where there is not a long track record of safe, attuned, and restorative communication, there is a certain degree of uncertainty about what their "next move" will be at any given moment. This will keep our senses on alert for threat detection, and because of the bias toward negative information, there may be a narrowing of attention or inaccurate estimation of specific features or frequencies of the other person that indicate an intention of rejection or harm. If our mood and expectations are negative, our field of attention may narrow in specific ways [FREDERICKSON2005]. A positive state, on the other hand, can help broaden our attentional spotlight and increase our access to a wider thought-action repertoire [FREDERICKSON2005].

In fact, people with anxiety disorders have a general tendency toward selective attention bias toward threatening stimuli [FORCELLI2017]. For example, people with spider phobias have a lower decision threshold for determining if a shape is a spider [WEIERICH2015], overestimate the speed of spider stimuli moving toward them [BASANOVIC2019], as well as overestimate the size of real-life spiders [SHIBAN2016]. Some studies using computational evidence suggest that attentional biases toward threats may be associated with enhanced learning about aversive stimuli [WISE2019]. Moreover, brain imaging studies reveal increased connectivity between various regions in people with attentional biases toward negative information.

For example:

■ People with spider phobia show greater connectivity between the pulvinar and amygdala than people without spider phobia [NAKATAKI2017].

■ People with social anxiety disorder show greater connectivity between the pulvinar and the visual and frontal cortices while viewing faces [TADAYONNEJAD2016].

■ Women with posttraumatic stress disorder (PTSD), which is associated with hypervigilant attentional bias to threat, show greater blood oxygen signals (BOLD) in the Superior Colliculus (SC), Periqueductal Grey area (PAG) and locus coeruleus and increased functional connectivity between the SC and cingulate cortex, insula, and amygdala, while viewing faces [STEUWE2012].

The above studies suggest that there may be an exaggeration of threatening stimuli in people with a greater attentional bias toward threat [MCFADYEN2020]. Threatening stimuli can include animal categories such as spiders and snakes, as well as social cues such as various facial expressions. A person's attentional biases may lead them to misperceive, exaggerate or hold attention longer on negative facial cues and lead to aberrant threat processing as well as irritability and anxiety [HARREWIJN2021]. This bias may lead to defensive behaviors that are a mismatch to the situation.

Negativity biases affect how we communicate and respond to others and negatively impact our emotion regulation abilities and overall mental health and well-being. As mentioned earlier, our past experiences play a role in these predictive biases. Our prior expectations may exaggerate or misperceive what is occurring, as seen in the over-expectancy of threat in anxiety disorders [AUE2015]. When sensory input is unreliable, such as when it is impaired by attentional filtering, the brain-body uses estimates of the world based on previous experiences [MCFADYEN2020]. Negativity bias has been shown to play a role in anxiety, depression, posttraumatic stress disorder, and schizophrenia [SHOOK2007; HARREWIJN2021]. Another disadvantage of exaggerated threat detection is that some areas of the prefrontal cortex become hypoactive under threat and uncertainty. This hypoactive state disinhibits sympathoexcitatory circuits to help the brain-body system mobilize and organize a response that does not include the delays and inhibitions that comes from the more deliberate and conscious guidance of the prefrontal cortex [THAYER2009]. If there is prolonged prefrontal inactivity, this can lead to neural activations dominated by hypervigilance and perseveration [THAYER2009]. All of these create significant challenges in adapting to situations with sensitivity to context. Suppose a person experiences these biases toward negative and threatening stimuli and responds to situations with vigilance and defensiveness. In that case, it becomes difficult to increase their repertoire of strategies for response. This then robs their problem-solving algorithms of the data it could use to cease ineffective strategies and experiment with new ones (e.g., try out a behavior that is in response to a safe social interaction and monitor the results of that type of interaction).

Limited Data Means Less Accurate Algorithms

These predictive mechanisms can be beneficial or detrimental, depending on our first experiences. We can look at how this can hurt or harm a brain by looking at the time and space horizons of brain development. On the time horizon, the most explosive experience-dependent growth in the human brain is from the moment we leave the womb until we are about 3 years old [HARVARDDC1]. This 0-3 timeline is important to highlight because it signifies the time period where we are least in control of what surrounds us. We are least in control of the space that surrounds us (which includes environmental conditions and people).

On the space horizon, if we zoom out to look at a human as a node that builds off of the information of other nodes, we can see that, for the most part, 0-3 years will have the fewest interacting nodes communicating with it. Because our brain-body is so dependent on its experiences to build its networks, action patterns may occur when we were young that helped us survive the dynamics of our family of origin. These may not be patterns that are adaptive for all future relationships: they served as a minimum viable strategy in response to what was going on around us and the abilities or limitations of our caregivers. Those adapting methods were based on whatever our brain-body had access to in terms of data. Because we are only surrounded by a few people regularly for the first year of our life, our algorithms about how the "world works" are based on the data we get from a limited number of people over and over again. This is important for us to understand as we look at how we build predictive algorithms for social interactions:

Limited data means narrower representations of people and the world: Our brain uses statistical probabilities and deductive reasoning formulas to attempt to navigate and manipulate the world for survival and thriving. It uses whatever data it receives to create its predictions and reasoning.

- A smaller sample size means that our conclusions may not be reliable or valid (something that can hold its explanatory power in multiple situations).

- The repetitiveness of interactions means an over abundance of certain patterns. Because our brain-body uses experience to build many of its networks, if an experience, type of interaction, or environmental condition occurs regularly, it feeds data into the system to predict what things are most likely to occur.

This means that what happens to us during those years plays an important part in the predictions and paradigms our brain-body creates to help us adapt to what our particular environment and social systems have in store for us. These predictions get updated throughout life; however, because our existence is so fragile when we are young, our interactions in our first years teeter on a balance between life-threatening or life-enhancing. In our first phases of life, what our caregivers do to, with, and for us can be the basis of life or death. They hold our life in their hands. Because the information of how to navigate those particular people—who hold our life in their hands—is so critical, many resources are devoted to deciphering, predicting, and storing every move they make, every tiny piece of information that could help or harm us, or that we could ignore. Those tiny pieces of information come in the form of frequencies from their body—smell, heat, pressure, pitch, volume of sounds, speed of movement, to name a few. The trial-and-error process of learning to detect and react to those frequencies and signals becomes part of our neural and behavioral survival repertoire. Anything that relates to such a deep sense of life enhancement or life depletion is something the brain-body holds as *the* highest priority for us to pay attention to. Our attentional mechanisms become your protection.

When we first arrive in this world, we have no choice over who is there and what awaits us. What we pay attention to helps our brain-body system navigate and manipulate the surroundings and people who are there. This forms the basis of much of our neural architecture that we then carry with us as we explore new terrains and interact with new people. These experiences can have permanent effects on how patterns of information we perceive are processed and used to make personal meaning out of signals coming from social interactions [SCHORE1994]. The experience-dependent nature of the orbitofrontal system means that its ability to enhance sensitivities and inform our brain-body system as to how to act and what to do in social situations is highly connected to our past [DEECKE1985].

To understand human communication, it is helpful to understand how many unconscious, nonverbal processes occur as we detect and analyze incoming socioaffective stimuli. Developmental neuroscience asserts that due to how interactions are processed and how much they are influenced by our early experiences, humans form biases or tendencies toward certain emotional responses [EMDE1983] and that certain neurophysiological and neuroanatomical circuits become more readily activated than others based on earlier experiences [MALATESTA1989]. These more readily activated circuits bias the infant's evaluation of novel situations and stimuli even before the brain has fully processed the incoming information [TRONICK1986]

This means that a powerful system exists within us that influences the sequence of movements we generate in response to what we are sensing in our social interactions. This system is occurring at an unconscious level and is based on a limited data set from the few people we were surrounded with when we first came into the world. Our sense of self is an accumulated database of our social experiences. It uses deduction and predictions based on past social interactions to fill the gaps in our current and future social experiences. Because of this, the gaps, misunderstandings, and distortions that influence our self-understandings also filter how we attempt to understand other minds [DEHAENE2010]. These unconscious processes pose a big challenge to our communication skills. Because our brain is building many of its networks and predictive algorithms from the moment we are born, and we only have a certain number of people we interact with during those years, the sequence of movements and internal states we have with them become the basis of how we will detect and respond to stimuli for the rest of our lives. Without being aware that these automated reaction sequences and expectations are occurring, it is difficult to change them. Once something is implicitly stored, it is activated and not easily deleted or changed [CRITCHLEY2013].

CHAPTER SUMMARY

These gaps, shortcuts, and unconscious influences are important to remember as we continue to explore the various mechanisms, strategies, and ways humans communicate. In many of our interactions, we risk a distortion between what we desire as an outcome of our social exchanges and the signals we send out to others, as well as what we perceive from them. We may think we are responding to others' signals in ways that are accurate and complete pictures of what is going on internally for them; however, science points to the fact that much of what we are perceiving is distorted by systems that are pre-emptively and unconsciously operating and directing our sensory and processing systems to pay attention and make meaning of what we perceive based on our first exchanges with caregivers. Communication can be a source of challenge and unnecessary stress due to these implicit, unconscious processes. However, attuned communication and expression are also our greatest tools for regulating our nervous systems and balancing challenge and restoration. Our best chance at updating our responses so that they are not simply automated reactions based on our past is to make them accessible to our conscious awareness. To do that, we must move them from the unconscious into what Stanislas Dehaene calls the conscious workspace [DEHAENE2010]. We can become more conscious of these forces by learning about our unconscious processes and the many influences that enter our behaviors and communication patterns. As we do that, we begin to create a shared language and understanding that we can access consciously. This is a step toward using communication as a tool for regulation. In the next chapters, we will continue to explore regulation as one of the foundations of communication and how attunement and biobehavioral mechanisms help us achieve our goals through communicative interactions.

REFERENCES

[AHERN1991] Ahern, G. L., et al. (1991). Right hemisphere advantage for evaluating emotional facial expression, *Cortex, 27,* 193–202.

[AUE2015] Aue, T., & Okron-Singer, H. (2015). Expectancy biases in fear and anxiety and their link to biases in attention. *Clinical Psychology Review, 42,* 83–95.

[BASANOVIC2019] Basanovic, J., Dean, L. Riskind, J. H., & MacLeaod, C. (2019). High spider-fearful and low spider-fearful individuals differentially perceive the speed of approaching, but no receding, spider stimuli. *Cognitive Therapy and Research, 43,* 514–521.

[BERNSTON1994] Berntson, G. G., Cacioppo, J. T., Quigley, K. S., & Fabro, V. T. (1994). Autonomic space and psychophysiological response. *Psychophysiology,* 31, 44–61.

[BONANNO2001] Bonanno, G. A. (2001). The self-regulation of emotion. In T. J. Mayne & G. A. Bonanno (Eds.), *Emotions: Current Issues and Future Directions* (pp. 251–285). New York, NY: Guilford Press.

[BONANNO2013] Bonanno, G. A., & Burton, C. L. (2013). Regulatory flexibility: an individual differences perspective on coping and emotion regulation, *Perspectives on Psychological Science.*

[BONANNOKELTNER1997] Bonanno, G. A., & Keltner, D. (1997). Facial expressions of emotion and the course of conjugal bereavement. *Journal of Abnormal Psychology, 106*, 126–137.

[BOVIN2008] Bovin, M. J., Jager-Hyman, S., Gold, S. D., Marx, B. P., & Sloan, D. M. (2008). Tonic immobility mediates the influence of peritraumatic fear and perceived inescapability on posttraumatic stress symptom severity among sexual assault survivors. *J. Trauma. Stress, 21*, 402–409. 10.1002/jts.20354

[CACIOPPO1999] Cacioppo, J. T., Gardner, W. L., & Berntson, G. G. (1999). The affect system has parallel and integrative processing components: Form follows function. *Journal of Personality and Social Psychology, 76*, 839–855.

[CAMERON2001] Cameron, O.G. (2001) *Visceral Sensory Neuroscience: Interoception.* Oxford University Press, New York.

[COIFMAN2010] Coifman, K. G., & Bonanno, G. A. (2010). When distress does not become depression: Emotion context sensitivity and adjustment to bereavement. *Journal of Abnormal Psychology, 119*, 479–490. doi:10.1037/a0020113

[COLE1994] Cole, P. M. Mi chel, M. K., & Teti, L. O. (1994). The development of emotion regulation and dysregulation: A clinical perspective. *Monographs of the Society for Research in Child Development, 59*, 73-100.

[COLE1992] Cole, P. M., & Zahn-Waxler, C. (1992). Emotional dysregulation in disruptive behavior disorders. In D. C. S. L. Toth (Ed.), *Developmental Perspectives on Depression* (pp. 173–209). Rochester, NY: University of Rochester Press

[COTE2005] Côté, S. (2005). A social interaction model of the effects of emotion regulation on work strain. *Academy of Management Review, 30*, 509–530. doi:10.2307/20159142

[CRITCHLEY2013] Critchley, H. D. (2013). Visceral influences on brain and behavior. *Neuron, 77*, 624–638. doi: 10.1016/j.neuron.2013.02.008

[CUNNINGHAM2008] Cunningham, W. A., van Bavel, J. J., & Johnsen, I. R. (2008). Affective flexibility: evaluative processing goals shape amygdala activity. *Psychological Science 19*, 152–160.

[DAMASIO1994] Damasio, A. (1994) *Descartes' Error*. New York: Grosset/Putnam.

[DAMASIO1995] Damasio, A. (1995). Toward a neurobiology of emotion and feeling: Operational concepts and hypotheses. *The Neuroscientist, 1*, 19–25.

[DANIELS2021] Daniels, S. et al. (2021) Effects of inescapable stress on responses to social incentive stimuli and modulation by escitalopram. *Psychopharmacology, 238*, 3239–3247.

[DEECKE1985] Deecke, L., et al. (1985). Timing function of the frontal cortex in sequential motor and learning tasks. *Human Neurobiology, 4*, 143–154.

[DEHAENE2010] Dehaene, S. (2010). *Consciousness and the Brain: Deciphering How the Brain Codes Our Thoughts*. New York, New York: Viking Press.

[DEW2011] Dew, T. Z., & Cabeza, R. (2011). The porous boundaries between explicit and implicit memory: behavioral and neural evidence. *Annals of the New York Academy of Sciences, 1224*, 174–190.

[EIDELMAN2016] Eidelman-Rothman, M., et al. (2016). Prior exposure to extreme pain alters neural responses to pain in others. *Cognitive, Affective & Behavioral Neuroscience, 16*, 662–671.

[EISENBERG1995] Eisenberg, L. (1995). The social construction of the human brain. *American Journal of Psychiatry, 152*, 1563–1575.

[EMDE1983] Emde, R. N. (1983). The pre-representational self and its affective core. *Psychoanalytic Study of the Child, 38*, 165–192.

[ETCOFF1984] Etcoff, N. L. (1984). Selective attention to facial identity and facial emotion. *Neuropsychologia, 22*, 281–295.

[ETKIN2004] Etkin, et al. (2004). Individual differences in trait anxiety predict the response of the basolateral amygdala to unconsciously processed fearful faces, *Neuron, 44*, 1043–1055.

[EVERLY2013] Everly, G. S., & Lating, J. M. (2013). *A Clinical Guide to the Treatment of the Human Stress Response,* 3rd ed. New York, NY: Springer.

[FOLKMAN2000] Folkman, S., & Moskowitz, J. T. (2000). Positive affect and the other side of coping. *American Psychologist, 55,* 647–654. doi:10.1037/0003-066X.55.6.647

[FORCELLI2017] Forcelli, P. A., Waguspack, H. F., & Malkova, L. (2017). Defensive vocalizations and motor asymmetry triggered by disinhibition of the periaqueductal gray in non-human primates. *Frontiers in Neuroscience 11,* 163.

[FREDERICKSON2005] Fredrickson, B. L., & Branigan, C. (2005). Positive emotions broaden the scope of attention and thought–action repertoires. *Cognition and Emotion, 19,* 313–332. doi: 10.1080/02699930441000238

[FREEMAN1942] Freeman, G. L., & Pathman, J. H. (1942). The relation of overt muscular discharge to physiological recovery from experimentally induced displacement. *The Journal of Experimental Psychology, 30,* 161–174.

[GEHRICKE2000] Gehricke, J.-G., & Shapiro, D. (2000). Reduced facial expression and social context in major depression: Discrepancies between facial muscle activity and self-reported emotion. *Psychiatry Research, 95,* 157–167. Retrieved from *http://www.sciencedirect.com/science/article/ pii/ S0165178100001682*

[GELLHORN1956] Gellhorn, E. (1956). Analysis of autonomic hypothalamic functions in the intact organism. *Neurology, 6,* 335–343.

[GELLHORN1967] Gellhorn, E. (1967). *Principles of Autonomic-Somatic Integrations: Physiological Basis and Psychological and Clinical Implications.* Minneapolis, MN: University of Minnesota Press.

[GELLHORN1970] Gellhorn, E. (1970). The emotions and the ergotropic and trophotropic systems. *Psychologische Forschung, 34,* 48–66. *https://doi.org/10.1007/BF00422862*

[GOLDSMITH2004] Goldsmith, H. H., & Davidson, R. J. (2004). Disambiguating the components of emotion regulation. *Child Development, 75,* 361–365. doi:10.2307/3696643

[HARVARDDC1] Harvard Center on the Developing Child, Experience Builds Brain Architecture: *https://developingchild.harvard.edu/science/ key-concepts/brain-architecture/*

[HOVDESTAD1996] Hovdestad, W. E., & Kristiansen, C. M. (1996). Mind meets body: on the nature of recovered memories of trauma. Women Ther. 19, 31–45

[JOHNSEN1991] Johnsen, B. H., & HUgdahl, K. (1991). Hemispheric asymmetry in conditioning to facial emotional expression. *Psychopathology*, *28*, 154-162.

[KARATSOREOS2013] Karatsoreos, I. N. (2013). Resilience and vulnerability–a neurobiological perspective. *F1000Prime Reports*, *5*, 13. doi: 10.12703/P5-13

[KATO2012] Kato, T. (2012). Development of the coping flexibility scale: evidence for the coping flexibility hypothesis. *Journal of Counseling Psychology*, *59*, 262–273. doi:10.1037/a00 27770

[KELTNER1993] Keltner, D., Ellsworth, P. C., & Edwards, K. (1993). Beyond simple pessimism: Effects of sadness and anger on social perception. *Journal of Personality and Social Psychology*, *64*, 740–752.

[KNIGHT1999] Knight, R., Staines, W., Swick, D., & Chao, L. (1999). Prefrontal cortex regulates inhibition and excitation in distributed neural networks. *Acta Psychologica*, *101*, 159–178.

[LARSON2007] Larson, C. L., Nitschke, J. B., & Davidson, R. J. (2007). Common and distinct patterns of affective response in dimensions of anxiety and depression. *Emotion*, *7*, 182–191. doi:10.1037/1528-3542.7.1.182

[LAZARUS1984] Lazarus, R. S., & Folkman, S. (1984). *Stress, Appraisal, and Coping*. New York, NY: Springer.

[LEDOUX1996] LeDoux, J. (1996). *The Emotional Brain*. New York: Simon and Schuster.

[LEDOUX2001] LeDoux, J. E., & Gorman, J. M. (2001). A call to action: overcoming anxiety through active coping. *The American Journal of Psychiatry*, *158*, 1953–1955. doi: 10.1176/appi.ajp.158.12.1953

[LEVINE1977] Levine, P. A. (1977). *Accumulated Stress, Reserve Capacity and Disease*. Ann Arbor, MI: University of California, Berkeley.

[LUPIEN2006] Lupien, S. J., Ouellet-Morin, I., Hupbach, A., Tu, M. T., Buss, C., Walker, D., et al. (2006). Beyond the stress concept: allostatic load-a developmental biological and cognitive perspective, in *Developmental Psychopathology, Vol. 2: Developmental Neuroscience* (2nd Ed.), eds Cicchetti D., Cohen D. J. (pp. 578–628). Hoboken, NJ: John Wiley & Sons.

[LUETHI2008] Luethi, M., Meier, B., & Sandi, C. (2008). Stress effects on working memory, explicit memory, and implicit memory for neutral and emotional stimuli in healthy men. *Frontiers in Behavioral Neuroscience, 2*, 5. doi: 10.3389/neuro.08. 005.2008

[MALATESTA1989] Malatesta, C. Z. et al., (1989). The development of emotion expression during the first two years of life. *Monographs of the Society for Research in Child Development, 54*, 1–103.

[MANDLER1966] Mandler, G., & Watson, D. L. (1966). Anxiety and the interruption of behavior. *Anxiety and Behavior.* In Spielberger C. (Ed.), Anxiety and behavior. New York: Academic Press,. 263–288.

[MARX2008] Marx, B. P., Forsyth, J. P., Gallup, G. G., & Fusé, T. (2008). Tonic immobility as an evolved predator defense: implications for sexual assault survivors. *Journal of Clinical Psychology, 15*, 74–90. doi: 10.1111/j.1468-2850.2008.00112.x

[MCEWEN2007] McEwen, B.S., Wingfield, J.C. (2007). Allostasis and Allostatic Load*, Editor(s): George Fink, *Encyclopedia of Stress* (Second Edition), Academic Press, 2007, Pages 135-141, *https://doi.org/10.1016/B978-012373947-6.00025-8.*

[MCEWEN2010] McEwen, B. S., & Wingfield, J. C. (2010). What's in a name? Integrating homeostasis, allostasis and stress, *Hormones and Behavior, 57 (2):105-11*

[MCFADYEN2020] McFadyen, J., Dolan, R. & Garrido, M.I. (2020). The influence of subcortical shortcuts on disordered sensory and cognitive processing, *Nature Reviews Neuroscience, 21*, 264–276.

[MEICHENBAUM1985] Meichenbaum D. (1985). *Stress Inoculation Training: A preventative and treatment approach;* New York: Pergamon Press; pp. 120–39.

[NAKATAKI2017] Nakataki, M. et al. (2017). Glucocorticoid administration improves aberrant fear-processing networks in spider phobia. *Neuropsychopharmacology, 42*, 485–494.

[NAUTA1982] Nauta, W. J. H., & Domesick, V. B. (1982). Neural associations of the limbic system. In A. L. Beckman (Ed.), *The Neural Basis of Behavior* (pp. 175–206). New York: SP Medical and Scientific Books.

[NIJENHUIS1998] Nijenhuis, E. R., Vanderlinden, J., & Spinhoven, P. (1998). Animal defensive reactions as a model for trauma-induced dissociative reactions. *Journal of Traumatic Stress 11*, 243–260.

[ORANGE2011] Orange, D. M. (2011). Speaking the unspeakable: "the implicit," traumatic living memory, and the dialogue of metaphors. *International Journal of Psychoanalytic Self Psychology, 6*, 187–206. doi: 10.1080/15551024.2011.552171

[PANDYA1985] Pandya, D. N., & Yeteria, E. H. (1985). Architecture and connections of cortical association areas. In A. Peters & E. G. Jones (Eds.), *Cerebral Cortex: Vol. 4. Association and Auditory Cortices* (pp. 3–61). New York: Plenum.

[PATON2006] Paton, J. F., Nalivaiko, E., Boscan, P., & Pickering, A. E. (2006). Reflexly evoked coactivation of cardiac vagal and sympathetic motor outflows: observations and functional implications. *Clinical and Experimental Pharmacology and Physiology, 33*, 1245–1250. doi: 10.1111/j.1440-1681.2006.04518.x

[PAYNE2015] Payne, P., & Crane-Godreau, M. A. (2015). The preparatory set: a novel approach to understanding stress, trauma, and the bodymind therapies. *Frontiers in Neuroscience, 9*, 178.

[PAYNE2015A] Payne, P., Levine, P. A., & Crane-Godreau, M. A. (2015). Somatic experiencing: using interoception and proprioception as core elements of trauma therapy, *Frontiers in Psychology, 6*, 423.

[PORGES2004] Porges, S. W. (2004). Neuroception: a subconscious system for detecting threats and safety. *Zero to Three, 24*, 19–24.

[PRIBRAM1991] Pribram, K. H. (1991). *Brain and Perception: Holonomy and Structure in Figural Processing*. Hillsdale NJ: Erlbaum.

[ROEDIGER1990] Roediger, H. L. (1990). Implicit memory: retention without remembering. *American Psychologist, 45*, 1043.

[ROTTENBERG2004] Rottenberg, J., & Gotlib, I. H. (2004). Socioemotional functioning in depression. In *Mood disorders* (pp. 61–77). John Wiley & Sons. Retrieved from *http://dx.doi.org/10.1002/9780470696385.ch4*

[ROTTENBERG2005] Rottenberg, J., Gross, J. J., & Gotlib, I. H. (2005). Emotion context insensitivity in major depressive disorder. *Journal of Abnormal Psychology, 114*, 627–639. doi:10.1037/0021-843X.114.4.627

[RYAN1997] Ryan, R. M., Kuhl, J. & Deci, E. L. (1997) Nature and autonomy: An organizational view of social and neurobiological aspects of self-regulation in behavior and development. *Development and Psychopathology, 9*, 701–728.

[SCHERER2009] Scherer, K. R. (2009). Emotions are emergent processes: They require a dynamic computational architecture. *Philosophical Transactions of the Royal Society B: Biological Sciences, 364*, 3459–3474.

[SCHORE1994] Schore, A. (1994) *Affect Regulation and the Origin of the Self: The Neurobiology of Emotional Development.* Hillsdale, NJ: Erlbaum.

[SHEPPES2012] Sheppes, G., Scheibe, S., Suri, G., Radu, P., Blechert, J., & Gross, J. J. (2012). Emotion Regulation choice: A conceptual framework and supporting evidence. *Journal of Experimental Psychology: General.* Advance online publication. doi:10.1037/a0030831

[SHIBAN2016] Shiban, Y., et al. (2016). Treatment effect on biases in size estimation in spider phobia. *Biological Psychology, 121*, 146–152.

[SHOOK2007a] Shook, N. J., Fazio, R. H., & Vasey, M. W. (2007a). Negativity bias in attitude learning: a possible indicator of vulnerability to emotional disorders? *Journal of Behavior Therapy and Experimental Psychiatry, 38*, 144–155.

[SHOOK2007b] Shook, N. J., Pena, P., Fazio, R. H., Sollers, J. J., & Thayer, J. F. (2007b). Friend or foe: heart rate variability and the negativity bias in learning about novel objects. *Psychophysiology, 44*, S39.

[STEUWE2012] Steuwe, C. et al. (2012). Effect of direct eye contact in PTSD related to interpersonal trauma: an fMRI study of activation of an innate alarm system. *Social Cognitive and Affective Neuroscience, 9*, 88–97.

[TADAYONNEJAD2016] Tadayonnejad, R., Klumpp, H., Ajilore, O., Leow, A., & Phan, K. L. (2016). Aberrant pulvinar effective connectivity in generalized social anxiety disorder. *Medicine, 95*, e5358.

[THAYER2009] Thayer, J. F., & Lane, R. D. (2009). Claude Bernard and the heart-brain connection: Further elaboration of a model of neurovisceral integration, *Neuroscience and Biobehavioral Review, 33*, 81–88.

[THAYER2005] Thayer, J. F., & Lane, R. D. (2005). The importance of inhibition in dynamical systems models of emotion and neurobiology. *Brain and Behavioral Sciences, 28*, 218–219.

[THAYER2004] Thayer, J. F., & Friedman, B. H. (2004). A neurovisceral integration model of health disparities in aging. In: Anderson, N. B., Bulato, R. A., & Cohen, B. (Eds.), *Critical Perspectives on Racial and Ethnic Differences in Health in Late Life* (pp. 567–603). The National Academies Press, Washington, DC.

[TRONICK1986] Tronick, E. Z., Cohn, J., & Shea, E. (1986). The transfer of affect between mothers and infants. In T. B. Brazelton & M. W. Yogman (Eds.), *Affective Development in Infancy* (pp. 11–25). Norwood, NJ: Ablex.

[WEIERICH2015] Weierich, M. R., & Treat, T. A. (2015). Mechanisms of visual threat detection in specific phobia. *Cognition and Emotion, 29*, 992–1006.

[WILLINGHAM1989] Willingham, D., Nissen, M., & Bullemer, P. (1989). On the development of procedural knowledge. *Journal of Experimental Psychology: Learning, Memory, and Cognition, 15*, 1047–1060. *http:// dx.doi.org/10.1037/0278-7393.15.6.1047*

[WISE2019] Wise, T., Michely, J., Daya, P., & Dolan, R. J. (2019). A computational account of threat-related attentional bias. *PLoS Computational Biology, 15*, e10007341.

[WU2013] Wu, G., Feder, A., Cohen, H., Kim, J. J., Calderon, S., Charney, D. S., et al. (2013). Understanding resilience. *Frontiers in Behavioral Neuroscience, 7*, 10. doi: 10.3389/fnbeh.2013.00010

3

COMMUNICATION AS A FORM OF FEEDBACK RESPONSIVENESS, BIOBEHAVIORAL ATTUNEMENT, AND ATTACHMENT

What is it that gives us a sense that we are safe and cared for within a relationship? When someone seems to be present and attuned to what you are saying or the nonverbal signals you are sending out, how does this affect your internal state and communication behaviors with that person? In the previous two chapters, we saw that communication is a feedback tool that can be used to help us regulate our nervous systems as well as navigate and manipulate our environment particularly when we are young and have less mastery over our brain-body systems. We saw that our earliest socio-communicative experiences begin to build neural circuitry that supports self-regulating mechanisms within us. We also learned that nonverbal and verbal signals make up the serve-and-return exchanges that are critical to building internal architecture needed for optimal brain development, optimized functioning, and basic survival. In this chapter, we will continue our focus on the use of communication as a means of nervous system regulation, survival, and optimization through the lens of attachment theory and biobehavioral attunement.

Before we discuss attachment and attunement, let us return to a systems-thinking perspective as we explore the idea of communication. An important element of systems thinking is to reflect on the function and goal of a system as a way to understand its behaviors. The concept of whether something is achieving what we are trying to do is tied to "effectiveness." If something is effective, it answers our question of "is it working?" To follow up on that question, we must also ask what we are in fact trying to do. If we are not clear on that, the question of "is it working" is irrelevant. We may also end up using ways to assess progress using misguided measures. As an analogy, if we want to determine if a home heating and cooling system is working and we only look at a specific temperature on the thermostat to determine this, we may miss assessing other aspects related to what the system is actually designed to do. For example, if we determine that the heating and cooling system has a goal of keeping people comfortable, as well as using energy efficiently to keep costs low, we may look to other assessment measures that go beyond just the temperature on the thermometer, such as insulation, window thickness, and other criteria. In the same way, when we think about effective communication, we need to determine its goal. Since, at our most fundamental level, we are always aiming to achieve homeostasis, one way we can assess whether communication is effective is to explore whether it is assisting with our homeostatic regulatory processes. The more efficiently communication assists us with maintaining homeostasis, the more we can categorize it as effective in achieving its goal. When communication moves us away from using energy efficiently to survive and flourish, it means that communication is now an obstruction of our most basic, life-driving goals.

The goal of homeostasis has within it the goal of energy conservation—not expending unnecessary energy that can be used for repair and maintenance. Because homeostasis is also tied to thriving, it also includes the criteria of energy surplus, finding ways to free up energy available for work toward future projection [DAMASIO2018]. Because of this, the underlying goal of communication is to optimize our energy processes in order to:

- Extract resources from the external environment to maintain homeostasis in the form of food, water, shelter, and social support.

- To regulate our internal state so that energy and resources can be used for future planning and prevention of future tissue damage.

Integrating these ideas together leads us to two key questions for exploring effective communication:

- What internal state does the communicator want to achieve?

- What internal state and corresponding behaviors does that same communicator want to initiate in the other person?

The answers to both of these questions are dynamic and constantly changing as each signal gets transmitted and received by both parties. An example of a desired internal state for a communicator will relate to their current energy levels and what they are trying to achieve. For example, if they are feeling overwhelmed and that a situation is demanding more of their cognitive resources than they are currently capable of accessing, their desired state may be to feel less challenged, less overwhelmed. In that case, they may want a quieter interaction and environment, with fewer decisions to make, and fewer stimuli to respond to. By contrast, if someone has experienced recent isolation, low energy, boredom, or withdrawal from activities that challenge them in healthy ways, their goal during an interaction may relate to initiating higher levels of excitatory and mobilizing types of energy and behavior. This ties back to the concept of regulatory flexibility from Chapter 2. Our ability to maintain homeostasis lies in the idea that it is not one or more particular strategies. Flexibility itself *is* a type of strategy, rather than any specific action or sequence of actions. The idea of a strategy being inherently adaptive or maladaptive is known as the fallacy of uniform efficacy, which highlights that the most resilient individuals have high degrees of inconsistency and variability when it comes to strategies used for self-regulation because they are dynamically and responsively updating their behaviors in response to emerging details of each situation [BURTON2016; FOLKMAN2004]. Returning to the analogy of the thermostat and heating and cooling system, a thermostat at 70 degrees Fahrenheit may not always be the optimal temperature for achieving the goal of people feeling comfortable and keeping costs down. They may want cooler on some days, or warmer on others. In this sense, communication is a way of sending signals out according to our continuously fluctuating relationships and responses to our environment, and both internal and external stimuli. All of these contribute to changes in a person's physiology, which also changes their goals and preferences in each situation. If a person is calm and feels comfortable and satisfied, and then the next moment an interaction they have with someone sparks an increase in their fight or flight response, their goal becomes significantly different. This changes how they will use their communication and behavior.

Because of that, the ability to attune and flexibly respond to signals is paramount to more or less all human behavior and communication. We see this idea reflected in developmental brain research, where interactions between the newborn and the mother are seen as regulators of internal homeostasis [OVTSCHAROFF2001]. Within that context of interactive homeostatic regulation, attachment theory offers a useful framework. While we have touched on attachment theory in previous chapters, we will go more into it in detail here.

ATTACHMENT THEORY IS IN FACT "REGULATION THEORY"

Although attachment theory was traditionally emphasized in the field of behavior and emotion, there is now enough support from bodily-based, physiological research on interactive regulatory processes that attachment theory can also be called "regulation theory" [SCHORE2008]. As already discussed in previous chapters, because of how brains mature over time, the infant or young child does not have access to self-regulating features [SCHORE2008; HARVARD2023]. It must outsource these to an attachment figure. This is a nonnegotiable aspect of being human (and applies more generally to all mammals). The interdisciplinary developmental and neurobiological research that has spanned over the past couple of decades since the emergence of attachment theory's core idea reveals that the relationships and emotional transactions with primary attachment figures early in life impact the maturation of brain systems involved in affect and self-regulation throughout the lifespan [SCHORE2008].

So What Is Attachment Theory?

As described in Chapters 1 and 2, the primary role of a caregiver—which we will now call an attachment figure—is to attune to the dynamic shifts in the child's body-based states of arousal. As the child's brain and nervous system are still in the early phases of development and not yet mature enough for the child to independently regulate their internal state, such as the ability to minimize excitatory activity when they are getting over-aroused, the attachment relationship helps mediate the child's regulating mechanisms to engage in social activity, play, exploration, as well as recovery periods of disengagement. With the help of these sequences of engagement, disengagement, attunement, misattunement, and re-attunement, an infant increases its abilities to self-regulate and become a more independent, self-reliant, and internally resourceful person [MAHLER1975]. In this sense, emotions and affective states are initially regulated by others, but as the infant's neurophysiology complexifies and matures, the child is increasingly more capable of self-regulating. Self-regulation includes the ability to flexibly regulate one's own internal state in contexts where they are alone, as well as in interconnected contexts and interaction with others [FELDMAN2012]. While the origins of attachment theory focused on child-caregiver regulation, research has emerged over the past few decades in the field of adult attachment behaviors, including how these can be affected by our early childhood experiences.

Indeed, developmental researchers propose that interactive homeostatic regulation between members of dyads is a pillar of all intimate relationships from infancy to adulthood [PIPP1987]. In this book, we will explore both the child-adult aspects of attachment as well as how attachment and interactive regulation theory influence communication between adults. The term attachment figure generally refers to a child's caregivers, whereas in adult attachment theory, attachment figures can be significant others such as spouses. Much of adult attachment research is focused on intimate and romantic relationships as these tend to reflect the concept of dependence most closely on a primary figure.

Secure and Insecure Attachment

Attachment theory also includes the concepts of secure versus insecure attachment. On a broad level, secure attachment is tied to sensitive and responsive attunement to the dynamic, emergent verbal and nonverbal signals of another person. This system of attunement is connected to the oxytocin system and helps create bonding behaviors within human relationships. According to Feldman and colleagues, oxytocin-releasing behavioral and bonding mechanisms can get disrupted when an attachment figure, such as a parent or caregiver, is unable to properly attune to the signals occurring within the dyad. This inability can be related to mental health challenges such as depression, anxiety, and addiction, as well as physical illness, absence due to work, distraction, and other behavioral issues that may stem from adverse childhood experiences and posttraumatic stress [FELDMAN2012]. When a person is misattuned, unavailable, or threatening, this inhibits the microbehaviors and signals that lead to the release of oxytocin. These kinds of disruptions within early attachment experiences can influence behaviors that continue into adult relationships and can play a role in insecure attachment patterns [HAZAN1994]. In this chapter, we will look at how attunement and responsiveness principles lead to effective communication in terms of their ability to regulate homeostatic processes.

EFFECTIVE COMMUNICATION IS AN ONGOING PROCESS OF FEEDBACK RESPONSIVENESS

Communication is a tool for enhancing our ability to maintain homeostasis. The more we understand this, the more we can assess what our system needs in order to use communication as a tool to achieve this. Two mechanisms are critical for this type of effective communication:

- The ability to express our internal state and intention to another as accurately as possible to help us achieve homeostasis. To repeat, homeostasis is tied to the maintenance of internal systems, avoidance of external threats, and projection into the future.

- The ability to understand the internal state and intentions of the person we are communicating with in order to know our best next action.

These two mechanisms stem from a concept known as *biobehavioral synchrony*—a concept within the field of affiliative neuroscience.

Biobehavioral Synchrony: An Emphasis on Bottom-Up, Clearly Observable Patterns

The study of behavioral synchrony brings an emphasis to bottom-up, clearly observable, and temporally organized patterns of micro-level social signals [FELDMAN2012]. This viewpoint was brought about by one of the original attachment researchers, John Bowlby, who shifted the study and exploration of behavior from psychoanalytic theory to the concrete assessment and meticulous documentation of behavior in natural ecologies of daily routines and moment-to-moment observations [FELDMAN2012]. This is crucially important as we discuss communication, which involves both verbal and nonverbal signals. These signals are mechanically produced into something perceivable by another—that is precisely what makes it a form of communication. Because of this, communication *is* behavior. It is a set of behaviors with specific goals, intensities, frequencies, and durations. Although the behaviors that form communication are influenced by the internal physiology of a person and their mental state, the actual micro-signals that can be picked up by human sensory receptors are the only phenomena that are available to another person. Most attachment research focuses on these micro-behaviors between parent and child; however, continuously emerging research affirms similar patterns of synchrony within friendships and romantic bonds. By understanding the micro-behaviors of bond formation, we get a sense of how communication assists in the goal of homeostatic regulation (and all of its related components such as goal achievement, sense of safety, belonging, etc.). As Feldman's research suggests, the study of attachment and affiliation is about synchronous behavioral exchanges between one person's internal physiological systems and mental states and how these impact micro-level behaviors that organize the bonding process in dyads [FELDMAN2012].

While we continue to explore communication as behavior across the lifespan, we see that the communication patterns between parent and infant play a particular role in revealing the importance of heightened attunement to the signals of each person. During the first phases of life, communication is critical to the infant's survival. Research demonstrates that in fact, during periods of bond formation, a biobehavioral reorganization occurs: the parents' physiology and behavior reflect a heightened sensitivity to infant cues, which prepares them for the task of caring for the infant with reliance only on micro-signals [FELDMAN2012]. As the parents and child continue to accumulate sequences of behaviors together in serve-and-return feedback exchanges, they become sensitive to the physiology and behavior of each other, particularly to the intensity, rhythms, and temporal qualities of these cues [FLEMING1999].

The coordination of movements and behavior reflects an ongoing feedback mechanism between each person's ongoing physiology and outwardly expressed communication and behavior. Early attachment research highlights the importance of an infant experiencing synchrony during their earliest experiences in order to support brain and behavior maturation, the ability to handle stress, and the child's lifetime capacity for social affiliation—which forms the foundation for their future parenting abilities [MEANEY2010]. As infants grow and become increasingly more active participants in their social world, their experience with affective matching is important for their development and predicts various aspects of childhood and adolescent social behavior, including moral orientation, self-regulation, competent social skills, and attachment security [FELDMAN2007]. Research has also shown that maternal and paternal roles follow distinct patterns of synchrony: maternal synchrony tends to be more socially oriented and cyclic. In contrast, paternal synchrony has a stronger focus on the environment and exploration [FELDMAN2003]. During the preverbal phase, synchrony is based on nonverbal patterns of expression of internal states. As symbolic thought and language develop, synchrony develops along two parallel tracks: one nonverbal line that maintains the dyad-specific patterns of affect synchrony involving nonverbal coordination of gaze, vocal quality, and facial expressions, and the second track of verbal coordination that consists of levels of empathy and self-disclosure [FELDMAN2012; FELDMAN2007b]. This research supports the idea that affect synchrony (attunement of each person's affective state) is a biological mechanism that continues throughout the lifespan and is found in interactions between parents and adolescents, close friendships, and romantic partnerships [FELDMAN2012]. Affect synchrony is supported by three key biological mechanisms [FELDMAN2012]:

- Autonomic reactivity

- Affiliative hormones

- Brain activation

Autonomic Reactivity and Vagal Tone

Cardiac vagal tone is an index that measures the respiratory cycle by quantifying rhythms of the heart and reveals the degree of a person's parasympathetic regulatory activity [PORGES2022]. Studies on cardiac vagal tone show that rhythms between caregiver and child are interrelated, suggesting that parasympathetic control during social interactions is part of a co-regulatory process [FELDMAN2010]. Vagal tone is tied to the functioning of the vagus nerve, a large cranial nerve originating in the brainstem that connects visceral organs to the brain. The parasympathetic nervous system is deeply intertwined with the vagus nerve due to most of the neural pathways of the parasympathetic system traveling through it [PORGES2022]. The vagus nerve contains both motor (efferent) fibers and sensory (afferent) fibers[1] [PORGES2022]. The motor fibers of the vagus nerve influence the functioning of the visceral organs, which include the digestive organs, heart, and deep layers of the skin. Humans, as well as other mammals, have two distinct vagal circuits:

- An unmyelinated circuit that originates in the dorsal motor nucleus of the vagus. The unmyelinated motor pathways of this system are found in most vertebrates and support neural regulation of subdiaphragmatic organs (internal organs below the diaphragm) [PORGES2022].

- A myelinated circuit that originates in an area of the brainstem called the nucleus ambiguus. This myelinated circuit is uniquely mammalian and helps regulate supradiaphragmatic (above the diaphragm) organs such as

---

[1] Motor fibers are nerve fibers that carry signals from the central nervous system (brain and spine) to the muscles of the body, including smooth (involuntary) and skeletal (voluntary) muscles. Smooth muscles are part of the autonomic nervous system and are found in the walls of hollow organs, such as in the walls of blood vessels, the stomach, intestines, veins, gastrointestinal tract and respiratory tract [BIGA2019]. Skeletal muscles are voluntary muscles that generally work with tendons to pull on bones and are part of the somatic nervous system.

the heart and lungs. It does this by functioning as a brake on the heart that can rapidly inhibit or disinhibit vagal tone to the heart to either immobilize and calm or mobilize an individual [PORGES2022].

Studies show that when mothers and infants engage in affect synchrony, heart-rate coupling is significantly higher than nonsynchronous interactions [FELDMAN2011A]. Research suggests that although much of mammalian biological synchrony is based on touch, such as licking and grooming, human biological synchrony can be influenced through voice, facial expression, and ongoing micro-behaviors (FELDMAN2011A). Indeed, the vagus nerve and its heart-brain connections during social interactions also connect to systems that influence facial expression, voice, and the ability to listen to someone speaking. We will go further into these specific mechanisms in Chapter 6.

Affiliative Hormones and Brain Activation

The neuropeptide oxytocin (OT) plays an important role in the formation of mammalian bonds and helps to reduce stress, enhance social competence, and cultivate social affiliation throughout the lifespan [WEAVER2004; FRANCIS2002]. In mammals, oxytocin-dependent affiliation networks and stress management systems are influenced by caregiver proximity and behavior, such as licking and grooming [MEANEY2010]. For example, studies have shown that young mammals who receive more grooming and touch [MEANEY2010]:

- Exhibited higher OT receptor densities in brain areas related to social affiliation.

- Showed more benefits from enriched environments.

- Were better able to handle stress.

- Offered more optimal parenting behaviors to their own offspring [CHAMPAGNE2008; CHAMPAGNE2007].

The majority of research on OT within human attachment processes has primarily focused on plasma OT (pOT) [FELDMAN2007]. In studies measuring OT from early pregnancy to postpartum, pOT levels remained stable within each mother and predicted the amount of eye gaze, "motherese" vocalizations, positive affect, and affectionate touch the mother engaged in toward the infant [FELDMAN2007]. Mothers with secure attachment profiles showed increased pOT after mother-infant interactions and stronger activations in brain areas that are rich in OT receptors [STRATHEARN2009].

In adults, higher pOT levels are linked with bonding processes throughout life, including more optimal bonding to one's own parents [GORDON2008] and secure attachment within romantic partnerships [TOPS2007]. A study involving mothers and daughters and a stressful event showed that Urinary OT (uOT) increased after a mother-daughter conversation following the stressful event [SELTZER2010]. Increases in pOT have also been shown in correlation to nonverbal displays of romantic love [GONZAGA2006]. Salivary OT (sOT) levels also show links with social affiliative behaviors. Levels of sOT have been shown to increase:

- Immediately before breastfeeding [WHITE-TRAUT2009].
- After massage in adults [CARTER2007].
- Following touch-related couples therapies [HOLT-LUNSTAD2008].
- Following parent-infant interactions with high levels of touch (not in interactions with low levels of tactile contact) [FELDMAN2010].

Oxytocin is shown to play a dual role in both bonding *and* reducing stress in humans and other mammals [HEINRICHS2007; NEUMANN2008]. Various studies suggest various mechanisms by which OT has anxiolytic (anxiety-reducing) effects:

- Increasing activity of emotion and cognitive processing areas of the brain while reducing neural activity in areas related to controlling visceral and autonomic responses [FEBO2009].
- Influencing the release of serotonin [YOSHIDA2009].
- Playing a role in variations in the OT receptor gene in regulating anxiety [COSTA2009].

Across mammalian species, bonds between infants and caregivers and bonds between adult reproductive partners show parallels in the psychoneuroendocrine mechanisms of coregulation [CARTER1998; HENNESSY1997]. This co-regulating mechanism lies within the core of the hypothalamic–pituitary–adrenal axis (HPA) and the autonomic nervous system. The primary function of this regulating system is to upregulate the system in order for the organism to take action to deal with a potential threat, and then to downregulate the system to maintain homeostasis once the threat is over [HAZAN2006]. Research on married couples has shown a regulating effect on partners physiology such as blood pressure. In one study, where each partner wore ambulatory devices to measure their blood pressure throughout the day and used time-stamped journal entries to show when they had interactions with their partner, blood pressure was significantly lower when the partner was present, compared to when they had one-on-one interactions with others, or when they were alone [GUMP2007].

Oxytocin and Gender

Studies on the relationship between OT and its effects on stress have revealed some contradictions: some report links between OT and *higher* levels of cortisol, which can be an indicator of increased stress response [MARAZATTI2006]. By contrast, other studies show correlations between OT and lower stress levels [HEINRICHS2007]. Some researchers suggest that the mixed findings are due to gender-specific differences in the effects of OT on stress and that early-rearing experiences influence the oxytocin system in sexually dimorphic ways[2]. Some of these gender-specific effects include:

- In animal studies on anxiety, OT manipulations showed different effects in females and males [SLATTERY2010].

- OT was shown to be related to relationship distress in women but not in men [SLATTERY2010].

- Links between OT and stress are tighter in females, which has led to the theory that women use social bonds for the management of stress [TAYLOR2000]. This may be linked to OTs role as a signal to the mother for regulating stress and maintaining close attachment bonds [FELDMAN2012].

LACK OF BIOBEHAVIORAL SYNCHRONY

The still-face paradigm is an important framework for understanding how lack of responsiveness in nonverbal communication plays a role in stress levels and social dynamics. The study was designed by Tronick and colleagues in the 1970s and has continued to be widely used in over 80 empirical studies, with robust findings regardless of variations such as infant gender and risk status [MESMAN2009]. The original research focused on mother-infant interactions and has since been expanded to include fathers and toddlers. The study

---

[2] Sexual dimorphism is a condition where the two sexes of the same species exhibit different characteristics beyond the differences in their sexual organs [BRITANNICA2022].

consists of a caregiver and infant sitting face-to-face and playing. The first phase has the parent engaging with their baby, smiling, and making sounds and movements in response to the baby's behaviors. In the second phase, the parent stops responding and engages in "still-face" for two minutes. After 2 minutes, the parent re-engages in a reunion or repair phase by responding normally with smiles, sounds, and movements. Meta-analyses of this experiment have shown that during the still-face period, infants show reduced positive affect and gaze, with increased negative affect, and also show a carry-over effect of this into the reunion/repair phase [MESMAN2009]. Higher levels of positive affect and lower negative in the infant during the still-face were also predictive of secure attachment at one year of age [MESMAN2009]. In other studies on cortisol and biobehavioral synchrony, Feldman and colleagues found concordance, following the still-face experiment, between mothers' and infants' cortisol levels, which correlated with mys-synchrony [FELDMAN2010]. This gives an indication as to how lack of responsiveness and nonverbal communication signals can affect parent-child stress levels.

This lack of responsiveness and its related stress levels give us clues as to how important attunement is within social communication. Significantly, longitudinal studies suggest that the synchronous experiences within parent-child dynamics transfer into other affiliative bonds throughout life [FELDMAN2012]. Interactions between romantic partners also parallel the underlying synchrony of the nonverbal and verbal lines and are related to the partners' vagus nerve functioning and oxytocin levels [FELDMAN2012]. What this tells us is that the synchronous patterns of nonverbal and verbal signals we co-create with others are part of a biological mechanism of nervous system functioning.

The biological importance of verbal and nonverbal synchrony is reflected in research that suggests that the absence or disruption of this synchrony is tied to dysregulation and impairments to social competencies and affiliative bonding. These studies form the basis of what is called high-risk parenting. In the following section, we will discuss some of the mechanisms associated with what is called high-risk parenting as a way to understand micro-level behaviors that form the basis of nonverbal communication. Although these studies focus on parent–child interactions, they are nonetheless useful for exploring how synchrony or lack of synchrony are affected by a person's internal state—and how this then influences another person's state and corresponding behaviors. Moreover, as we will see in some of this research, the effects of biobehavioral patterns in childhood can have enduring impacts on our ability to attune and create affiliative bonds later in life. It can be helpful to keep in mind that as we communicate with experience-dependent brain-body systems, we may be expecting and seeking signals and communication patterns in another person that may not be as natural for them based on their attachment history, as well as other factors that can influence these micro-behaviors.

High-Risk Parenting

High-risk parenting is associated with parental behavior that is misattuned to the child's. This can be in the form of excessive behavior (intrusiveness) or lack of responsiveness. Most studies on high-risk parenting have focused on maternal behavior, but some studies, such as the still-face paradigm, have begun to incorporate more exploration of father and other caregiver behaviors [FELDMAN2003]. Studies by Feldman and colleagues have found links between excessive maternal behavior and maternal anxiety and minimal maternal behavior with maternal depression [FELDMAN2009]. These behaviors are observable and measurable: for example, mothers diagnosed with clinical depression take five times longer than controls to engage in their first episode of synchronized eye gaze with their infant, and the intervals between episodes of joint social engagement are seven times longer than controls and engage in temporal patterns of inactivity, flat affect, and minimal contact [FELDMAN2012]. Maternal anxiety, on the other hand, is associated with a pace that is three and half times faster than controls and associated with misattuned responses, where the infant signals a need for rest, but the mother engages in arousal-inducing parenting [FELDMAN2012]. This reflects the pattern of intrusive parenting reported by Alan Schore in *Affect Regulation and the Origins of the Self* [SCHORE1994].

Moreover, the patterns of depressed mothers, including less social behavior, withdrawal, declined physical proximity, and low levels of coordinated nonverbal and verbal behavior, were shown to persist over time [FELDMAN2012]. Children of these mothers showed reduced symbolic complexity and play that was characterized by repetitive functional activities [FELDMAN2012]. Although the children of depressed mothers are at greater risk of psychiatric disorders, research on family systems suggests that more involved and synchronous fathering can moderate the effects of maternal depression [FELDMAN2007A]. This offers clues, once again, that the more opportunities humans have to engage in biobehavioral synchrony and form affiliative bonds, the more likely they are to benefit from its protective factors in stress regulation and optimized brain functioning.

Other Factors That Can Influence Biobehavioral Patterns

While this book will not cover all the factors that can lead to variations in biobehavioral patterns, certain conditions are worth noting briefly. One of these is premature birth, which can influence synchrony and attunement because it is also associated with over-stimulatory parenting [FELDMAN2006]. In the context of the vagus nerve and its associated social engagement system, premature infants often have disruptions to their abilities to send clear social messages, which in turn makes interactions challenging and anxiety-producing for caregivers. This may then lead to intrusive tactics, particularly if there are other health or developmental challenges [FELDMAN2006].

Studies in biobehavioral synchrony show that it is universally optimal for interactions to be attuned to an infant's social behaviors and internal state, and not over-stimulating, while providing the infant containment [FELDMAN2012]. Nevertheless, research has shown that cultural differences may be linked with differences in parenting behaviors. For example, some studies suggest that parents in industrialized countries use more active forms of touch and present objects more than parents in nonindustrialized societies—where parents maintain closer physical proximity and engage in less active behavior [FELDMAN2006]. Some studies, such as those focused on Israeli and Palestinian families, also show that although the pathways to help infants attain developmental milestones may vary across cultures, the levels of self-regulation that are reported are similar across those cultures, which suggests that there many pathways to the same goal of interactive regulation [FELDMAN2006].

CHAPTER SUMMARY

In this chapter, we explored communication as a tool for achieving homeostasis through social behaviors. Elements of maintaining and achieving homeostasis include using sociality as a means to extract resources efficiently, protect against real and present threats, and engage in biobehavioral synchrony to enhance regulation and restoration of internal systems. By bringing the ultimate goal of communication to the forefront, we are better able to assess whether it is effective. Within this exploration, we saw that communication is a behavior and is a dynamic feedback process that is tied with affiliative hormones such as oxytocin and biobehavioral patterns of responsiveness and attunement to the internal state of oneself and another person. We also looked at how a lack of this responsiveness can influence the regulation of another person's nervous system. In the following chapters, we will dive deeper into the concept of communication as an energy-optimizer as well as face-voice-heart mechanisms used in communication and feedback, and processes related to the translation of kinesthetic, sensory, visceral signals into symbols, and language.

REFERENCES

[BIGA2019] Biga, L. M., Dawon, S., Hardwell, A., Hopkins, R., Kaufmann, J., LeMaster, M., Matern, P., Morrison-Graham, K., Quick, D., & Runyeon, J. (2019). *Anatomy & Physiology.* Oregon State University (*https://openstax.org/details/books/ anatomy-and-physiology*)

[BRITANNICA2022] Britannica, The Editors of Encyclopaedia. "sexual dimorphism". *Encyclopedia Britannica*, 23 Dec. 2022, *https://www.britannica.com/science/sexual-dimorphism*. Accessed 13 February 2023.

[BURTON2016] Burton, C. L., & Bonanno, G. A. (2016). Regulatory flexibility and its role in adaptation to aversive events throughout the lifespan. In A. D. Ong & C. E. Löckenhoff (Eds.), *Emotion, Aging, and Health,* American Psychological Association: Washington DC (pp. 71–94).

[CARTER1998] Carter, C. S. (1998). Neuroendocrine perspectives on social attachment and love. *Psychoneuroendocrinology, 23*, 779-818.

[CHAMPAGNE2007] Champagne, F. A., & Meaney, M. J. (2007). Transgenerational effects of social environment on variations in maternal care and behavioral response to novelty. *Behavioral Neuroscience, 121*(6), 1353–1363.

[CHAMPAGNE2008] Champagne, D. L., Bagot, R. C., van Hasselt, F., Ramakers, G., Meaney, M. J., de Kloet, E. R., Joels, M., & Krugers, H. (2008). Maternal care and hippocampal plasticity: evidence for experience-dependent structural plasticity, altered synaptic functioning, and differential responsiveness to glucocorticoids and stress. *Journal of Neuroscience, 28*, 6037–6045.

[COSTA2009] Costa, B., Pini, S., Martini, C., Abelli, M., Gabelloni, P., Ciampi, O., Muti, M., Gesi, C., Lari, L., Cardini, A., Mucci, A., Bucci, P., Lucacchini, A., & Cassano, G.B. (2009). Mutation analysis of oxytocin gene in individuals with adult separation anxiety. *Psychiatry Research*, 168, 87–93.

[DAMASIO2018] Damasio, A R. (2018). *The Strange Order of Things. Life, Feeling, and the Making of Cultures*. New York: Pantheon Books.

[FEBO2009] Febo, M., Shields, J., Ferris, C. F., & King, J. A. (2009). Oxytocin modulates unconditioned fear response in lactating dams: an fMRI study. *Brain Research, 1302,* 183–193.

[FELDMAN003] Feldman, R. (2003). Infant-mother and infant-father synchrony: The coregulation of positive arousal. *Infant Mental Health Journal, 24,* 1–23.

[FELDMAN2006] Feldman, R., & Eidelman, A. I. (2006). Neonatal state organization, neuro-maturation, mother-infant relationship, and the cognitive development of small-for-gestational-age premature infants. *Pediatrics, 118,* e869–e878.

[FELDMAN2006] Feldman, R., Masalha, S., & Alony, D. (2006). Micro-regulatory patterns of family interactions; Cultural pathways to toddlers' self-regulation. *Journal of Family Psychology, 20,* 614–623.

[FELDMANWELLER2007] Feldman, R., Weller, A., Zagoory-Sharon, O., & Levine, A. (2007). Evidence for a neuroendocrinological foundation of human affiliation: plasma oxytocin levels across pregnancy and the postpartum period predict mother–infant bonding. *Psychological Science, 18,* 965–970.

[FELDMAN2007A] Feldman, R. (2007c). Maternal versus child's risk and the development of parent-infant and family relationships in five high-risk populations. *Development & Psychopathology, 19,* 293–312.

[FELDMAN2009] Feldman, R., & Eidelman, A. I. (2009a). Biological and environmental initial conditions shape the trajectories of cognitive and social-emotional development across the first five years of life. *Developmental Science, 12,* 194–200.

[FELDMAN2010] Feldman, R., Singer, M., & Zagoory, O. (2010). Touch attenuates infants' physiological reactivity to stress. *Developmental Science, 13*(2), 271–278.

[FELDMAN2011] Feldman, R., Gordon, I., Zagoory-Sharon, O. (2011). Maternal and paternal plasma, salivary, and urinary oxytocin and parent–infant synchrony: considering stress and affiliation components of human bonding. *Developmental Science 14:4* (2011), 752–761.

[FELDMAN2011A] Feldman, R., Magori-Cohen, R., Galili, G., Singer, M., & Louzoun, Y. (2011). Mother and infant coordinate heart rhythms through episodes of interaction synchrony. *Infant Behavior and Development, 34*(4), 569–577.

[FELDMAN2012] Feldman, R. (2012) Bio-behavioral synchrony: A model for integrating biological and microsocial behavioral processes in the study of parenting. *Parenting: Science and Practice, 12*(2–3), 154–164.

[FOLKMAN2004] Folkman, S., & Moskowitz, J. T. (2004). Coping: Pitfalls and promises. *Annual Review of Psychology, 55*, 745–774.

[FRANCIS2002] Francis, D. D., Young, L. J., Meaney, M. J., & Insel, T. R. (2002). Naturally occurring differences in maternal care are associated with the expression of oxytocin and vasopressin (V1a) receptors: gender differences. *Journal Neuroendocrinology, 14*, 349–353.

[GUMP2007] Gump, B. B., Polk, D. E., Kamarck, T. W., and Shiffman, S. M. (2001). Partner interactions are associated with reduced blood pressure in the natural environment: Ambulatory monitoring evidence from a healthy, multiethnic adult sample. *Psychosomatic Medicine, 63*, 423–433.

[HARVARD2023] Brain Architecture, Harvard Center on the Developing Child. *https://developingchild.harvard.edu/science/key-concepts/brain-architecture/*

[HAZAN2006]. Hazan, C., Campa, M., & Gur-Yaish, N. (2006). What is adult attachment? In M. Mikulincer & G.S. Goodman (Eds.), *Dynamics of Romantic Love: Attachment, Caregiving and Sex* (pp. 47–70). New York: Guilford Press.

[HAZAN1994] Hazan, C., & Shaver, P. R. (1994). Attachment as an organizational framework for research on close relationships. *Psychological Inquiry 1*(5), 1–22.

[HEINRICHS2007] Heinrichs, M., & Gaab, J. (2007). Neuroendocrine mechanisms of stress and social interaction: implications for mental disorders. *Current Opinion in Psychiatry, 20*, 158–162.

[HENNESSY1997] Hennessy, M. B. (1997). Hypothalamic-pituitary-adrenal responses to brief social separation. *Neuroscience and Biobehavioral Reviews, 21*, 11–29.

[MAHLER1975] Mahler, M. (1975). *The Psychological Birth of the Human Infant: Symbiosis and Individuation.* London: Routledge. DOI *https://doi.org/10.4324/9780429482915*

[MARAZATTI2006] Marazziti, D., Dell'Osso, B., Baroni, S., Mungai, F., Catena, M., Rucci, P., Albanese, F., Giannaccini, G., Betti, L., Fabbrini, L., Italiani, P., Del Debbio, A., Lucacchini, A., & Dell'Osso, L. (2006). A relationship between oxytocin and anxiety of romantic attachment. *Clinical Practice and Epidemiology in Mental Health, 2,* 28.

[MEANEY2010] Meaney, M. J. (2010). Epigenetics and the biological definition of gene · environment interactions. *Child Development, 81,* 41–79.

[MESMAN2009] Mesman, J., & van Ijzendoorn, M. H. (June 2009). The many faces of the Still-Face Paradigm: A review and meta-analysis. *Developmental Review, 29*(2), 120–162.

[NEUMANN2008] Neumann, I. D. (2008). Brain oxytocin: a key regulator of emotional and social behaviours in both females and males. *Journal of Neuroendocrinology, 20,* 858–865.

[PIPP1987] Pipp, S., & Harmon, R. J. (1987). Attachment as regulation: A commentary. *Child Development,* 58, 648–652.

[SCHORE1994] Schore, A. (1994) *Affect Regulation and the Origin of the Self: The Neurobiology of Emotional Development,* Hillsdale, NJ: Erlbaum.

[SCHORE2008] Schore, A. (2008). Effects of a secure attachment relationship on right brain development, affect regulation and infant mental health. Department of Psychiatry and Biobehavioral Sciences University of California at Los Angeles School of Medicine.

[YOSHIDA2009] Yoshida, M., Takayanagi, Y., Inoue, K., Kimura, T., Young, L. J., Onaka, T., & Nishimori, K. (2009). Evidence that oxytocin exerts anxiolytic effects via oxytocin receptor expressed in serotonergic neurons in mice. *Journal of Neuroscience, 29,* 2259–2271.

[WEAVER2004] Weaver, I.C., Cervoni, N., Champagne, F. A., D'Alessio, A.C., Sharma, S., Seckl, J. R., et al. (2004). Epigenetic programming by maternal behavior. *Nature Neuroscience, 7*(8), 847–854.

4

COMMUNICATION AS A BEHAVIORAL TRANSMITTER AND ENERGY OPTIMIZER

How does a person's posture, tone of voice, facial gestures, and words change when they feel unsafe? What are the mechanisms humans use to protect themselves from danger? How does threat and danger – whether perceived or real – change our communication patterns? On the other hand, what happens to a person's communication patterns and signals when they want someone to come closer? How do our signals induce a sense of protection or connection from others? The concept of danger, survival, and threat are at the core of many theories that we will explore in this chapter related to sociality, attachment, and energy optimization.

In the previous chapters, we looked at some of the biobehavioral mechanisms of attunement and communication as a means of promoting nervous system regulation and brain functioning. We also explored how flexibility, feedback, and the ability to monitor, cease, adjust, continue, or enhance strategies for maintaining homeostasis are important for resilience and system regulation. A system responds to the feedback it is getting in order to constantly make adjustments, but it can only make an adjustment to something that has already happened in the past. In terms of human communication, we need to understand that communication is an emergent process: each micromovement, each action we perform, is in response to something that has occurred. It is an ongoing dynamic process. Within that dynamic, emergent process, there is still an overall goal that each human, each self-regulating system, is trying to achieve. We have already looked at this goal as relating to homeostasis and internal state regulation. Through that lens, we will see how communication is a tool we use to enhance our social existence and achieve various subgoals—all of which at a very basic level are tied to the most essential goal of all: survival.

COMMUNICATION FOR SURVIVAL

At the core of all of it, we can say that the "goal" of all systems is to survive. Survival is both a process and the result of using energy to avoid entropy: to keep the atoms and molecules of our brain-body system together in a cohesive form. This form functions as a self-organizing system that can move, adjust and extract resources and energy from outside itself in order to release that energy within its own internal subsystems as a way to slow down its deterioration. Resisting entropy is the first level of what we are trying to do at all times. The mechanisms and all various subsystems that are nested within a human organism work together to keep the system intact.

We are not just a system—we are also complex adaptive systems. A few features define a complex adaptive system. First, the complexity of a system means that it is a dynamic network of interactions between diverse and specialized components, parts, or agents [RIDDER2017]. Second, its adaptive nature means that it is capable of being influenced by feedback and, therefore, evolves, mutates, and self-organizes according to constantly changing micro-events or collections of events. Complex adaptive systems also have some form of history or memory, which means their current behavior is influenced by their past [RIDDER2017]. Moreover, complex adaptive systems show the property of emergence, meaning that the behavior of the ensemble may not be predictable according to the behavior of the components [RIDDER2017]. This emergent and evolving behavior of a complex adaptive system, such as humans, requires constant monitoring and response to micro-events. Because we exist in a reality where other humans (among other complex adaptive systems) exist, one of the constantly changing sources of micro-events that we must monitor and respond to is humans. Applying this view of systems interacting with other systems, we can propose that the most basic function of communication is to enhance human systems' ability to survive and flourish. Communication is a feedback-response mechanism we use to monitor our environment to extract energy for maintaining the ongoing processes of the subsystems that keep us alive. We also use these mechanisms not only to extract energy and resources but to avoid anything that would lead to dissipation of the system.

Our very first glimpse of this in action is with the newborn parent dynamic. As we saw in Chapter 1, humans use vocalization and facial gestures as a serve-and-return feedback process to ensure that basic needs are met and to build systems in the brain and body that help an individual regulate their own internal environment. This basic communication-for-survival process is most obvious in newborns because they are not yet self-regulating or have the motor skills needed to fully navigate and extract resources from the environment or fend off danger. Although we get better at self-regulating as we get older, survival is still the underlying goal for all of our communication, regardless of age.

Survival for humans is incredibly complicated because of our extremely high degree of social interaction. To look at how we use communication to survive, we need to look at how social interactions can contribute to or threaten our survival. One aspect of this is on a physical level. Survival, at a bare minimum, means avoiding the disintegration of our cellular structures. On the most obvious level, this means avoiding anything that could puncture or harm the tissue or physical integrity of our body, skin, or organs, which could lead to bleeding, disease, infection, etc. Sources of tissue-damage danger would include animals and humans who could physically injure or harm us with weapons and self-defense mechanisms (venom, claws, teeth), illnesses, and viruses, as well as things like falling, accidents, and environmental dangers like bacteria, drought, starvation, excessive cold, and heat.

Tissue-damage danger is the most "expensive" of all the dangers we can encounter. The amount of energy that needs to be used to repair cells means that energy is not available for other functions. System preservation is the top priority. If the system dies, nothing else matters. So, from an energy-optimization perspective, avoiding tissue damage is a system's highest priority. When we are very young, we do not have all the data we need to know what can cause tissue damage. We use learning and social referencing as a way to avoid trial and error to figure out what might harm us. We also use cumulative knowledge, which can come in the form of language and graphics—such as books, art, and stories—to help us benefit from previous generations' experience with threats and survival. Communication is one of the tools we can use to avoid tissue damage. There are three key ways we use it in this way: one is to prevent proximity of a threat, another is to request proximity of a source of support, and the third is to organize behavior for threat-prevention.

Communication is a warning signal to attempt to prevent the physical proximity of a threat or predator

We see communication as a warning signal in various species. For example, a dog's bark is a way to create an audible frequency to activate an alert response in an unknown organism. This can serve as a warning to not approach further. Using this audible signal requires less energy expenditure than if the dog had to use its physical force to fight off a threat. A human can use shouting to do this. Visible signals would include hand gestures, body posture, and size. Facial expression can also be a visible warning signal, but because of the small size of facial muscles, this requires proximity for another person to see accurately. The use of these depends on what the person or animal is capable of in terms of their resources. For example, a dog may be smaller in size, so the use of sound will be something it resorts to more quickly than a large dog. Humans can also use visible symbols that are known to be understood by others as a warning that they will resort to aggression, such as a weapon or insignia. This only works, however, if the symbol is understood by the encroaching threat. For example, if a person presented a knife or gun to another species or a person who had no idea what it was, this would not serve as a visible warning. The same can be said for words. The word "stop" will only work if the other person understands what that collection of sounds symbolizes. As we will see in Chapter 6 when we discuss voice frequencies, the nonverbal parameters of voice serve an important communicative function in parallel with verbal cues.

Communication is an airborne signal to request help or support in the case of illness, distress, or injury

The sound frequency of vocalizations, namely separation-distress vocalization, is a communication mechanism for virtually all mammals [HOFER2010]. The maintenance of stable body temperature also has a connection with the particular vocal mechanism of crying. Various theories examine how the larynx has evolved across species over time, from a valve to protect airflow in early air-breathing fish to later adaptations that involve vocalizations [HOFER2010]. One of those functions was to help a mother accurately detect the state or condition of offspring from a distance, as well as locate them if they separated from the nest [HOFER2010]. In mammals, close proximity to the nest was critical for maintaining stable body temperature and vocalizations from offspring serve as a signal to mothers to retrieve them. Human infants' cries are at a particular frequency that leads to a distress response in a caregiver

[DUDEK2016]. This ensures that the caregiver will not ignore the cry and will do what it takes to attenuate it. These cries in mammals and humans are not only used for separation distress but also for requesting help for physical injury illness. Facial gestures and body movements can also serve this purpose. However, audible signals are the most efficient because they do not require another to be focused on the individual and can be perceived across longer distances than subtler visible signals like facial expressions. Large, exaggerated physical gestures could be seen across longer distances; however, this may not be possible in the case of someone who does not have the capacity to create these large gestures—either because they lack physical maturity or they are in pain or injured.

Communication to organize behavior against a threat

An example of using communication to organize or influence behavior to avoid danger or threat would be if you saw someone about to walk into a street and they were not looking in the direction of a car coming toward them. Using your physical body to alert them or move them out of the way would not be fast enough to help them avoid being hit. An audible signal such as yelling has a chance of traveling fast enough. Moreover, the vocalization of a conspecific has a specific frequency range to cut through background sounds and activate a 'listening response' in the other [PORGES2021]. This frequency range in humans for example, is between 20 and 20,000 hertz [ROSEN2011]. This range, combined with an acoustic masking system within the middle ear, allows us to hear a human's voice despite all the other sounds coming in [PORGES2021].

In primates, for example, we also see this way of using communication (in this case, it is vocalization) as a way to organize against a threat. This also requires that the group of primates are able to detect and understand each other's signals without necessarily alerting the predator as to their whereabouts. To do this, the listening mechanisms need to be sensitive to specific frequency ranges that other species are potentially not capable of detecting. One way mammals do this is through airborne sounds, such as vocalizations that reach frequencies that are not detectable by reptiles [HOFER2010]. Airborne sounds can be picked up by mammals through tiny ear bones and an extra set of sensory hair cells [HOFER2010]. These features allow conspecifics to signal to each other across distances in ways that they understand, without the need to move their bodies or create vibrations that could be detected by reptiles or other predators that are able to detect their location through body movement vibrations. We see this in the ultrasonic frequencies of many rodents, who vocalize within the range of 20 to 100 kHz [HOFER2010].

These are just a few examples of how we use communication to prevent tissue-damage danger to ourselves and others. We will explore the use of words in later chapters as well, but for now, we will keep the discussion to audible and visible signals created by facial gestures, vocalizations, and body and limb movements.

In addition to protecting against tissue damage caused by a predator or weapon, communication is also a tool for promoting internal conditions of an organism that are critical for survival. Homeostasis is the ability or tendency of a living organism, cell, or system to keep the conditions inside it within an optimal range despite any changes in the conditions around it. Anything that disrupts or impairs cellular functioning will disrupt homeostasis. Toxins, injuries, aggressions, and inadequate amounts of necessary vitamins, minerals, oxygen, and other molecules can all impair cellular functioning and can be caused by environmental factors. Allostatic load, which is the wear and tear on the body due to excessive stress, also affects cellular functioning. Homeostasis includes not only mere survival but also what Antonio Damasio proposes as flourishing and projection of life into the future [DAMASIO2018]. Mere survival means we do just enough to keep our physical systems running to keep us alive. Projection into the future includes the capacity to optimize our energy usage to restore and replenish our systems and also prepare, project, and set up future-oriented systems for continued survival, adaptation, and optimization. Homeostasis, therefore, includes both survival and optimization.

COMMUNICATION FOR ENERGY OPTIMIZATION

As we saw earlier, communication is one of the tools we use to avoid threats and injury. It is also something we use to extract resources and optimize energy usage. Optimization is important for us to understand in the realm of communication because of its ability to help us achieve a narrower range of ideal conditions. This means that communication is something we can use to create situations and systems in our life that can continuously serve our projection into the future. First, let's take a look at the idea of optimization from a more general viewpoint.

Optimization means we continuously move up the scale into a narrower range of ideal conditions for survival and flourishing. For example, if we were living in a desert, the lower, wider end of preferences would be not dying from heat and dehydration or predators. Moving up the scale could include not only not dying, but actually finding a way to be in a more comfortable temperature (according to the range that is within our natural system settings) most of the time. As humans, because of our generalized intelligence, we have the capacity, due to features of our brain as well as our fingers, hands, and upright posture, to find ways to achieve that narrower range of preference (in this case, a narrower range of temperature). We could do that by creating, for example, something to shield us from the sun. Optimization could also relate to how a person earns a living. The lower, wider end of the scale of preferences could look like merely having enough income to pay rent. Moving up that scale could include having a short commute and fewer hours. Moving up the scale narrows the range of preferences. It becomes more specific.

Often, when we really look at them, these narrower ranges of preferences are tied to energy expenditure. When we find ways to expend less energy on one set of systems needed to maintain homeostasis, we free up energy to use for other systems and optimizations. We see this concept play out in Maslow's hierarchy of needs [MASLOW1943]. At the widest, lowest level, we have basic systems for maintaining homeostasis, such as shelter, water, and food. Just enough environmental resources to stay within the ranges of what our cells need to function. As we move up the pyramid, we include the optimization of the systems below and add a new range of preferences.

Each of these new levels of preferences is also tied to different aspects of our brain and nervous system. As we move up these levels, more energy is needed to supply the brain and nerve cells that correspond with the increasing complexity of achieving those activities. For example, if a person were to stay immobile, curled up in a ball, there would be a certain number of calories needed for that simple activity. Calories are a form of energy held together in a specific formation that can be broken down by the body. As the packets of molecules are broken down, the energy released from that process can be used by other systems inside the body. If that person were to do any other activity, they would need more energy extracted from the environment (more calories). As we add movement to our activity, we increase the need for decision-making, which is a form of neural activity that also requires energy. Move this way or that, look here or there, approach, avoid, etc. Each decision requires cells and networks in the brain and body to communicate with each other to receive, process, and send instructions based on continuously new information from each new vantage point created by our movement. Each of these micro-decisions costs energy. To fire up those cells, energy is needed to open blood flow and change cell polarization for action potentials. What all this means is that:

1. With each movement we make, we need energy from our environment.

2. Moving in increasingly complex ways makes us better at adapting to our environment, but it also means we need more energy.

3. Our systems are designed to help us continuously adapt and, therefore to continuously seek to extract energy from our environment.

4. The more we optimize systems, the more efficiently we use the energy we extract from outside resources to maintain survival. This can allow for an excess of energy that can then be used to continuously optimize, adapt, and survive.

Now that we have an idea of how important optimization is, let's look at how we use communication to not only survive but to make our lives easier through an optimized state of functioning.

Human optimization through sociality

As discussed earlier, optimization is a way of using energy as efficiently as possible to achieve our goals. As a reminder, our ultimate goal is maintaining homeostasis, which includes survival and a process of finding and using energy to continue projection into the future. One way to use energy efficiently for this goal is to avoid tissue-damage danger. Tissue repair requires energy to restore and maintain the physical integrity of the organisms, which means less free energy for protection, planning, and projections to help us continue. From a systems perspective, avoiding damage, rather than tending to it, is an optimal use of energy. In order to maintain the existence of the system (fight entropy), we also need to extract resources from our environment. We need energy inputs. We get these by extracting energy from our environment, such as food and water. The less amount of energy we use to get these inputs and avoid tissue damage, the more energy can be used for planning and projecting into the future, which helps the system perpetuate. Optimizing is a way of using less energy to avoid damage and extract resources to create a surplus of energy that can be used to perpetuate into the future.

One way humans (as well as many other species) have optimized these processes is through sociality [SMELSER2001]. Sociality is a tendency to associate with or from groups. As we saw in the previous chapters, we use mechanisms such as off-loading or out-sourcing to help us with many aspects of our survival and self-regulation when we are infants. This use of dyads and groups helps us maintain an ideal temperature, stay safe, fed, and hydrated—all of which help free up energy for strengthening muscles and bones and creating brain-body connections for balance, locomotion, and new and more complex cognitive skills. The more our basic needs for survival are met, the more neural and energy resources can be used for optimizing mechanisms to navigate and manipulate our environment, such as creating tools, machines, and communication technologies.

COMMUNICATION AS A SOCIOBEHAVIORAL TRANSMITTER

To understand how communication is used in conjunction with sociality to help us survive, we will look at communication as a behavioral transmitter. As Stefan Brudzynski proposes, all modes of communication are, in a sense, behavioral initiators, modulators, or inhibitors depending on the context, which fulfills the criteria of the behavioral transmitter [BRUDZYNSKI2009]. In this chapter, we will focus on communication as a behavioral transmitter that we use to increase our ability to survive and optimize our abilities to adapt and project into the future. In particular, we will explore the various configurations of voice frequencies and facial muscles that contribute to communication as a behavioral transmitter.

So, what is a behavioral transmitter exactly? It begins with a relatively weak physical or chemical event or stimulus occurring with one organism [BRUDZYNSKI2010]. As the signal of this event is transmitted outside the organism, it is capable of inducing responses in another organism that cost (require) additional energy [BRUDZYNSKI2010]. If one organism's signals induce new activity in another organism's somatic, autonomic, and endocrine systems, as well as their central nervous system, this is a "costly" energetic response. This is because any initiation of activity requires energy. That energy will need to come from outside that organism in order to continuously maintain the integrity of the system. The idea of transmitter in terms of communication is analogous to what happens with neurotransmitters: as one neuron sends a signal to another, that neuron receives the signal in the form of neurotransmitter molecules that bind to its receptors. As this occurs, the receiving neuron utilizes energy—adenosine triphosphate (ATP)—in a response that has much higher output energy than the initial energy of the stimulus molecule

[BRUDZYNSKI2010]. In a behavioral transmitter, we are expanding this idea of signals from one entire organism, leading to the activation of an entire organism. In both situations, the initial signals—such as voice or facial muscle movements—can be received by specialized auditory and visual receptors by the receiving organism and can induce activity from the central nervous system and entire organism. This corresponds to the lock-and-key principle of neurotransmitters, where the transmitter—and communication signal—is the key and is capable of unlocking or initiating an amplified response when it is received by the other cell's or organism's receptors [BRUDZYNSKI2010].

Communication, as a behavioral transmitter, is therefore a tool we use to increase our chances of survival and optimization by inducing activity in another organism. Human communication is a mechanism that relies on signal transmission and reception from one person to another to achieve these goals. Most importantly, we must remember that communication—as a behavioral transmitter—is a form of control. As we transmit signals about our physiological state or intention, we are doing this to increase our chances of survival by attempting to induce physiological and behavioral changes in another human. This may include warding off a person to avoid tissue damage or to entice a person to behave in a way that will help us maintain homeostasis. Communication can be used for survival in the moment, where we want to avoid tissue damage danger, or it can be about survival from a long-term perspective. This includes building relationships, teams, organizations, families, etc. As we convey signals through our voice, face, body posture, hands, and language, we can induce state and behavior changes in another person in conjunction with our short- and long-term survival goals.

This signal transmission system allows us to extract resources, fend off danger and optimize our energy usage by coordinating our behaviors with one another. To help us understand how we use these mechanisms, we will explore theories related to attachment and social dynamics throughout the upcoming sections and chapters.

MODERN ATTACHMENT THEORY

We explore attachment theory in Chapter 3 and will continue to integrate it as a foundational concept within human communication theory. In Chapter 3, we looked at the concepts of secure and insecure attachment. In this chapter, we will look at additional theories and frameworks that have evolved from the original research on attachment by John Bowlby and Mary Ainsworth. John

Bowlby was a psychologist and psychoanalyst who first proposed attachment as a framework for understanding child-caregiver behavior dynamics [BOWLBY1982; BRETHERTON1992]. An important aspect of this theory is a child's need to have a strong bond or connection to at least one primary caregiver, particularly during stressful situations, in order for the child to have healthy development across the lifespan [ABRAMS2013]. Mary Ainsworth expanded on this theory to include the concept of a Secure Base: a familiar person to return to after exploration [BRETHERTON1992]. Ainsworth also highlighted patterns of attachment behaviors that included secure, avoidant, and anxious. These patterns have been expanded and modified to include a pattern of a fourth pattern called disorganized attachment [BRETHERTON1992]. Attachment theory has also been developed into much more complex theories and into adult attachment patterns [HAZAN1994].

Modern attachment theory is based on three principles:

1. Bonding is an intrinsic human need.

2. Humans use relationships to enhance vitality by regulating emotion and fear.

3. Attachment and bonding are conducive to adaptiveness and growth [JOHNSON2019].

Dynamic-Maturational Model of Attachment and Adaptation

An important model that has been developed to further understand how attachment relationships affect human development and functioning is the dynamic-maturational model of attachment and adaptation (DMM), developed by developmental psychologist Patricia McKinsey Crittenden and colleagues [CRITTENDEN2011]. The DMM has a particular focus on child-parent and reproductive couple relationships. Another major aspect of the DMM is its focus on danger and survival. Earlier theories, such as those proposed by William Blatz, proposed play and safety as the core of attachment, whereas Bowlby emphasized attachment about protection from danger [BOWLBY1982]. Crittenden maintained this focus that attachment strategies are developed primarily to identify and protect oneself from danger [CRITTENDEN2011].

In alignment with the idea that all of our behavior is for the purpose of maintaining homeostasis (which involves survival and projection into the future), the DMM proposes that the central motivations of behavior are the protection of self and progeny [BOWLBY1982] and to protect against isolation. Within that model, attachment is viewed as:

- A pattern of behavior in a relationship
- Pattern of processing information
- Strategy for identifying and responding to danger

Another extension of Bowlby's work that is outlined in the DMM is that attachment is also connected to information processing, particularly that in order to survive psychologically distressing and dangerous situations, a psychological defense mechanism is used to exclude information [BOWLBY1982]. This idea of self-protective strategies and patterns of information processing in the context of danger and survival are central to the DMM [CRITTENDEN2011].

Danger, Adaptation, and Maladaptation: An Information Processing Model of Attachment

Every exposure to danger gives the brain-body system information it can use to predict and prevent future dangers. To make these predictions, the brain-body system uses past data and transforms it into something to be used at the current moment in the form of thoughts and behaviors [SCHERER2009; SCHORE1994]. If the transformation of this data is erroneous or outdated, this is a maladaptive response to a current event. This would mean that a person's behavior and response to a current challenge is missing information or transforming the information in erroneous ways. This could include perceiving an actual danger that is not there and, in doing so, creating an actual threat. An illustration of this would be if someone gets cut off in traffic, and they transform this information into an interpretation of the driver as an aggressor or threat, which then leads them to get out of their car at the next stop light to threaten them back. What was possibly not an actual life-threatening situation has now escalated into becoming one. Another example would be *not* perceiving danger when it would be life-protecting to do so. This could include not defending ourselves or others against someone who is a threat or failing to take measures that could help prevent danger, injury, or illness in future situations, such as not taking precautionary steps for outdoor and sports activities, not enhancing immunity by eating poorly, not engaging in other protective activities like self-defense classes, or neglecting to teach children about various dangers and what to do in response. Being prepared and protecting ourselves and others from danger allows us to stay alive, as well as create new algorithms and protective working models that help propel development forward. Being prepared for and dealing appropriately with threats and challenges builds agency: it helps us build a track record and neural networks involved in adaptive and accurate foreseeing that we *can* protect ourselves both psychologically and physically. This knowledge builds confidence and expands our ability to take on challenges and explore new territories. We can build agency not only to prevent and protect ourselves from physical threats but social–emotional types of challenges as well. Attachment theory highlights the importance of protection against danger: secure attachment revolves around a sense of being protected against danger and threat, while a history of not being protected when we are young can lead to many different types of maladaptive responses. The DMM proposes that these maladaptive responses are related to errors in information processing across the lifespan and that these information processing errors involve shortcuts.

SHORTCUTS

Short cutting is a psychological mechanism of incomplete information processing, where there is some exclusion of relevant information and inclusion of irrelevant information [CRITTENDEN2011]. Biological shortcuts allow humans to perform "time-precious" actions such as avoiding harm by using immediate, rapid responses and bypassing the slower more complex processes that involve foresight and planning [MCFADYEN2020]. An example of a biological shortcut is when our muscles reflexively move our hand away from a hot stove before we even feel that it is hot. Subcortical areas are the first to receive sensory input about the external environment and enact an immediate reflexive response [KANAI2015]. Although research over the past couple of decades has shown dynamic functional interactions between subcortical shortcuts and whole-brain processing, the role of these dynamics in cognitive processing has been underemphasized, particularly as it relates to disrupted information processing [MCFADYEN2020]. While shortcuts serve important survival functions, they also result in outdated or maladaptive transformations of information in the face of danger, which can lead to challenges in behavior and communication.

The information processing model of attachment points to the fact that the brain, as an organ used to make predictions and initiate protective actions, is most vulnerable to error when it is immature [CRITTENDEN2011]. Because of lack of motor coordination, size and neural development involved in predicting and preventing future threats, infants must rely on their caregivers for protection from danger. If a child experiences danger without protection and comfort by caregivers, this puts the child outside of what is called their zone of proximal development (ZPD) [VYGOTSKY1978]. When something threatening happens, and the child is not comforted or protected, the infant must "cobble together a neural network to generate protective behavior" [CRITTENDENN2021]. The child has to work with what it has in terms of information and the ability to process and transform information. These shortcuts are tied to erroneous, omitted, or outdated information, and can lead to a spectrum of maladaptive behavior and even psychological trauma.

Information processing errors and their prolonged effects on behavior and mental health can also occur for events that happen at any point in life, such as tragedy and trauma during a person's adulthood. Any event that is outside an individual's zone of proximal development can lead to severe dysregulation, shortcuts, and enduring consequences. A zone of proximal development is tied to an ability to process information within the existing neural and behavioral capacities of an individual. This term is often applied in early childhood contexts because of a child's lack of self-regulating brain networks and developing muscular and motor control and coordination of their body. However, this term can also be applied to adults: if an event occurs, such as events that happen in war or natural disaster, it is possible that the challenges occurred without the individual being able to prevent or protect themselves and can therefore lead to a similar type of "cobbling together" and information processing errors.

Crittendenn and colleagues propose three main conditions where information processing about danger is insufficient [CRITTENDENN2011]:

- **Immaturity**: an immature brain that does not have the complex features needed to fully process information.

- **Imminent danger**: a danger that is so imminent that taking any time to process the information more fully could result in death (imminent danger).

- **Complex causation**: events where information or critical aspects of the event are not visible (complex causation).

In addition, if standards for behavior change as one enters a new context or gets older, a protective behavior that results from a psychological shortcut might become maladaptive [CRITTENDEN2011]. Within the DMM framework, these maladaptive responses may include paranoia, deception, compulsive caretaking, and many others. As we saw earlier in Chapter 2, a major aspect of adaptive behavior is regulatory flexibility. This flexibility requires context sensitivity, which is the ability to accurately appraise threat and opportunity. Short-cutting excludes relevant information—things like another person's perspective or other systems-related perspectives—and may include irrelevant information, such as narrowing focus on a particular detail to the exclusion of other information that may actually be more relevant for problem-solving or preventing harm. This kind of shortcutting emerges in various anxiety-related disorders and phobias.

Recent research has been exploring how early subcortical processing and reciprocal subcortical-cortical interactions contribute to behavior and high-level cognition—and how this may influence processing anomalies and behaviors related to clinical anxiety, phobias, and distractibility [MCFADYEN2020]. The recruitment of neural shortcuts can be viewed as adaptive when we are faced with an actual potential threat. For example, the sooner we can determine whether what we are seeing is a snake or a rope, the sooner we can initiate a life-saving response. However, when these shortcuts are overexerted or under-exerted, this can impair a person's ability to respond adaptively. People with a specific phobia, such as spiders, for example, exhibit heightened detection sensitivity and lower decision threshold for spider images shown among other images [WEIERICH2015]. People with a phobia of spiders also overestimate the speed of spider stimuli moving toward them versus away from them [BASANOVIC2019] and overestimate the size of real-life spiders [SHIBAN2016]. Interestingly, computational research also suggests that attentional biases toward threats are associated with enhanced learning about aversive stimuli [WISE2019].

What research on these shortcuts reveals is that there are various forms of distorted, omitted, or erroneous information processing that are occurring. Some research suggests that this may be related to how the brain and eyes interact to capture and allocate attention. For example, the superior colliculus (SC) directs eye movements toward salient visual stimuli [KRAUSLIS2013], while the pulvinar plays a role in regulating and allocating attention via visual coding and synchronization of cortical activity [SAALMANN2012]. Recent neuroimaging suggests a functional interplay between the SC and the pulvinar in biasing attention toward threat and leading to a bottom-up exaggeration of threatening stimuli in people with anxiety and other attentional biases to threat, such as in phobias [KOLLER2019; MCFADYEN2019; TADAYONNEJAD2016; STEUWE2012].

Importantly, this research on neural shortcuts highlights how subcortical circuits can play a significant role in human perception, decision-making, social interactions, and communications. They do this in two ways:

- Altering computation within subcortical areas. For example, with enhanced responses to threats in the pulvinar [LE2014] and lower decision thresholds for escape in the SC [EVANS2018]. These altered computations act as filters that influence the strength and quality of what we see and learn about the world [NIV2019].

- Gating or biasing information processing by influencing higher-order functions like attention and prediction [MCFADYEN2020; LIANG2015].

While subcortical shortcuts are necessary for defensive responses to imminent danger, the optimization of defensive behavior that may occur can have maladaptive effects as well. This contrast between adaptive and maladaptive mechanisms is a key component of the Dynamic-Maturational Model (DMM) and corresponds to our discussion in earlier chapters about regulatory flexibility and sensitivity to context. Maladaptive or adaptive strategies depend on how well the strategy fits the context [PEERY 2014]. This model highlights the importance of understanding how our early attachment experiences may have led to shortcuts that were adaptive to us when we were helpless and had no choice over who we sheltered with and depended on to survive, but that may not be as adaptive when used in adult relationships and by a person who is not as dependent on a caregiver for their survival and protection. Considering these mechanisms as protective can help us understand the challenges that occur in human-to-human communication and interaction.

Protective Strategies: overview of DMM categories

To build protective strategies, an individual uses information from the past to build predictions [CRITTENDEN2011]. Due to immature and emerging self-regulation mechanisms and motor control when we are young, our best self-protective strategy as children is to seek out protection from a grown-up. The protective attachment and comfort within a child-parent relationship leads to patterns in processing information that become the basis of the child's protection and comfort-seeking behavior, which then affects the parent's protective and comfort-giving behavior [CRITTENDENN2011]. Multiple attachment relationships and dynamics exist within each family, and these relationships compete, support, and change each other over time. By understanding this, we can see an array of many possible protective strategies that function to prevent rejection or attack or abandonment [CRITTENDENN2011].

In the DMM framework, strategies are associated with various behaviors and information processing. The spectrum of strategies is also associated with varying exposure to threats. In his model, the higher-numbered "A" and "C" strategies reflect "exposure to more severe, pervasive and deceptive danger" [CRITTENDENN2011]. This overview of potential patterns in strategies listed below is not meant to be exhaustive or a definitive description and explanation of behaviors that may emerge during interactions (which affect communication strategies); it is meant to simply show another perspective that emerged from attachment researchers' studies and observations.

The following are protective strategies, behaviors, and information processing within the DMM framework [CRITTENDENN2011].

B Strategies reflect an integration of logical and affective information. The behavior associated with B strategies is an ability to negotiate to resolve problems and communicate thoughts and feelings. The predictions made from cognitive and affective information are accurate [CRITTENDENN2011].

"A" Strategies are related to distorted cognition. They also range in how negative affect is integrated into information processing: from omitting negative affective information (the lower numbers) to omitting negative affect and falsifying positive affective information (middle numbers) all the way to denying negative affective information and using delusional positive affect within information processing [CRITTENDENN2011].

A Strategies include [CRITTENDENN2011]:

- Inhibited/socially facile: Strategies that focus on the positive in others and inhibit affect to avoid disputes.

- Compulsive caregiving: When a person uses behavior and expresses emotions in ways that they believe others desire, and care for others as a way to meet their own needs—even if this is at their own expense.

- Compulsive Performance: Relates to having perfectionistic and workaholic behaviors and preference for challenging tasks.

- Compulsive Promiscuity: Behaviors that bias the use of a positive appearance to engage the attention of others without close involvement.

- Compulsive Self-Reliance: Strategies associated with doing things on one's own, even if they are unpleasant or painful, and succeeding without anyone's help.

- Compulsive Idealizing: A person who uses these strategies distorts their perception of dangerous people or conditions by only perceiving and processing positive information. This can also include using religion, philosophy, or a "self-transcendent" mission to reframe distress.

- Selfless: These strategies result in someone readily accepting other people's negative judgments about them and experiencing conflict between their own feelings and what other people want.

"C" Strategies are associated with information processing that distorts negative affective information and relies on either omitted cognition (C1-4); a combination of omitted true cognition (actual, real data) and falsified cognition (C5-6); or combines denied true cognitive information and delusional cognition (C7-C8) [CRITTENDENN2011]. C strategies include [CRITTENDENN2011]:

- Threatening-Disarming: A person using these strategies emphasizes their own feelings and needs and warns of future problems as a way to engage others.

- Aggressive: Strategies related to heroic, protective behaviors during crises and are also often associated with disarming and charming types of behaviors.

- Feigned Helplessness: Strategies related to a strong desire for comfort that highlight a person's vulnerability while disguising their abilities and competence in an effort to engage others.

- Punitive: Punitive behaviors are often tied to asserting authority, using persuasive management, enlisting support, and procuring resources to meet group goals and protect the unit.

- Seductive: In order to elicit appeasing behavior from others, a person using these strategies will alternate between enticing (even sexualized) behaviors and bitter resentment. There is a strong strategic bias toward eliciting involvement from other people.

- Menacing: Behaviors are geared toward an aggressive stance and secretive plotting against many enemies and presumed threats.

- Paranoid: A person using these strategies seeks to control inexplicit dangers by suspecting everyone and has a strategic bias toward hiding anger while displaying fear.

The central pillar of the above strategies is that they are responses to danger, including perceived danger, and are, therefore, protective strategies [CRITTENDENN2011]. From this danger-centered attachment perspective, we understand that the mechanisms within our brain-body system are geared toward predicting and avoiding danger. These mechanisms include information processing, how memory from past events is stored and integrated, and our attentional mechanisms. All of these neural processes are influenced by experiences of danger, which can lead to distortions, omissions, and other erroneous processing that influences behavior and communication. Many of these protective strategies may have been adaptive to a certain degree and during certain events, particularly when we were small and helpless. However, as information is distorted, this can increase the chance of the behavior being maladaptive to the situation. This concept goes back to feedback responsiveness, which emphasizes the importance of context sensitivity, the ability to notice how our actions create feedback, and a willingness and ability to adjust continuously and dynamically, cease, enhance, or continue a strategy according to feedback. Having erroneous or distorted inputs and processing makes it difficult to accurately interpret the context and choose a response that fits the energy requirements of a situation.

CHAPTER SUMMARY

In summary, our main goal for all behavior—and therefore communication—is to maintain homeostasis. We do this by keeping the physical integrity of our body intact and using energy efficiently to avoid tissue damage and internal organ problems. We also use communication to optimize energy efficiency by exchanging signals between us and another conspecific to outsource what we may not be able to do for ourselves and to coordinate behavior to achieve goals, extract resources, and fend off danger. Danger, damage, and physical harm are the costliest in terms of overall and long-term energy efficiency. This is because resources in the form of nutrients, tools, equipment, or other people's behavior are needed to repair the system. Using energy to obtain those resources for repair means that energy cannot be used for longer-term projections, planning, and prevention of future threats. Danger is at the root of our attachment needs and protective strategies. The need to fend off and prevent threats can become maladaptive if early experiences and/or distortions and challenges in information processing. Distortions and subcortical shortcuts may lead a person to engage in behaviors that are not sensitive to context, particularly if the behavioral strategies are rooted in maladaptive child-caregiver dynamics and are now being used in adult relationships.

Now that we have explored communication as a behavioral transmitter that helps us find ways to achieve and maintain homeostasis, we will look at the specific biological mechanisms that help us transmit and detect signals within communicative interactions. In the following two chapters, we will look specifically at signals and configurations created by facial movements (including the eyes), and vocalizations, as well as the mechanisms we use to receive audible signals.

REFERENCES

[ABRAMS2013] Abrams, D. B., et al. (2013). *Attachment Theory. Encyclopedia of Behavioral Medicine* (pp. 149–155). New York, NY: Springer.

[BARBOT2018] Barbot, A. & Carrasco, M. (2018) Emotion and anxiety potentiate the way attention alters visual appearance. *Nature* (8), 5938. *https://doi.org/10.1038/s41598-018-23686-8*

[BOWLBY1982] Bowlby, John (1982). *Attachment and loss: Volume III: Loss, Sadness and Depression.* New York: Basic Books.

[BRETHERTON1992] Bretherton, I. (1992). The origins of attachment theory: John Bowlby and Mary Ainsworth, *Developmental Psychology, 28,* 759–775.

[BRUDZYNSKI2010] Brudzynski, S. M. (Ed.) (2010). *Handbook of Mammalian Vocalization: An Integrative Neuroscience Approach.* Academic Press, San Diego.

[CRITTENDEN2011] Crittenden, Patricia M., and Landini, Andrea (2011). *Assessing Adult Attachment: A Dynamic-Maturational Approach to Discourse Analysis.* New York: W. W. Norton & Company.

[DAMASIO2018] Damasio, A. R. (2018). *The Strange Order of Things. Life, Feeling, and the Making of Cultures.* New York: Pantheon Books.

[DUDEK2016] Dudek, J., Faress, A., Bornstein, M.H., and Haley, D.W. (2016). Infant Cries Rattle Adult Cognition. *PLoS One, 11*(5), e0154283. *https://doi.org/10.1371/journal.pone.0154283*

[HAZAN1994] Hazan, C., and Shaver, P.R. (1994). Attachment as an organizational framework for research on close relationships. *Psychological Inquiry, 5*, 1–22.

[HOFER2010] Hofer, M. A. (2010). Chapter 2.3: Evolution of the infant separation call: rodent ultrasonic vocalization. In *Handbook of Mammalian Vocalization: An Integrative Neuroscience Approach*, Brudzynski, S. M. (Ed.). San Diego: Academic Press.

[HOLMES2014] Holmes, Paul, and Farnfield, Steve (Eds.) (2014). *The Routledge Handbook of Attachment: Implications and Interventions*. New York: Routledge.

[JOHNSON2019]. Johnson, S.M. (2019). *Attachment Theory in Practice: Emotionally Focused Therapy (EFT) with Individuals, Couples and Families* (p. 5). New York: The Guildford Press.

[KOENIG2020] Koenig, J. (2020). Neurovisceral regulatory circuits of affective resilience in youth: Principal outline of a dynamic model of neurovisceral integration in development, *Psychophysiology* (57).

[MASLOW1943] Maslow, A. H. (1943). A theory of human motivation. *Psychological Review, 50*(4), 370–396. *https://doi.org/10.1037/h0054346*

[MATHER2011] Mather and Sutherland (2011). *Perspectives on Psychological Science, 6*(2): 114–133.

[MEADOWS2008] Meadows, D. (2008). *Thinking in Systems: A Primer*. Chelsea Green Publishing: White River Junction, VT.

[MCFADYEN2020] McFadyen, J., Dolan, R. J., and Garrido, M. I. (2020). The influence of subcortical shortcuts on disordered sensory and cognitive processing. *Nature Reviews Neuroscience, 21*, 264–276.

[PORGES2021] Porges, S. (2021). *Polyvagal Safety: Attachment, Communication, Self-Regulation* (pp. 73–77). New York: W. W. Norton & Company Inc.

[RIDDER2017] Ridder, D. D., Stöckl, T., To, W. T., Langguth, B., Vanneste, S. Chapter 7 - Noninvasive Transcranial Magnetic and Electrical Stimulation: Working Mechanisms, in *Rhythmic Stimulation Procedures in Neuromodulation.* (2017) Evans, J.R., Turner, R.P., (Eds), Academic Press, Pages 193-223,

[ROSANBALM2017] Rosanbalm, K. D., and Murray, D. W. (2017). "Caregiver Co-regulation Across Development: A Practice Brief" OPRE Brief #2017-80. Washington, DC: Office of Planning, Research, and Evaluation, Administration for Children and Families, US Department of Health and Human Services.

[ROSSING2007] Rossing, T. (2007). *Springer Handbook of Acoustics* (pp. 747, 748). New York: Springer.

[ROSS2021] Ross, E. D. (2021). Differential hemispheric lateralization of emotions and related display behaviors: emotion-type hypothesis. *Brain Sciences, 11,* 1034. *https:// doi.org/10.3390/brainsci11081034*

[SCHERER2009] Scherer, K. R. (2009). The dynamic architecture of emotion: Evidence for the component process model. *Cognition & Emotion (23),* 1307–1351.

[SCHORE1994] Schore, A. (1994) *Affect Regulation and the Origin of the Self: The Neurobiology of Emotional Development.* Hillsdale, NJ: Erlbaum.

[SMELSER2001] Smelser, Neil J., and Baltes, Paul B. (Eds.) (2001). *Evolution of Sociality. International Encyclopedia of the Social & Behavioral Sciences* (p. 14506). New York: Elsevier.

THE MECHANICS OF COMMUNICATION SIGNALS

What gives us a clue that someone is interested in what we are saying, or offended? What are we looking at in another person's face when we are having a conversation with them? Do we notice where our eyes go? Do we know what our facial expression looks like when we feel threatened, curious, or amused? In the previous chapters, we saw that communication is a feedback tool that can be used to help us regulate our nervous systems as well as navigate and manipulate our environment. We also saw that our earliest experiences contribute to self-regulating mechanisms within us and that information processing plays a role in our perception of others' verbal and nonverbal signals. In this chapter, we will focus on the mechanics of how some of these communicative signals are created, transmitted, and exchanged. As we continue to examine communication as a means of nervous system regulation, survival, and optimization, it is important to mention all the various forms of communication signals. These can include thermal, temperature changes, chemical, and olfactory, such as pheromones and smells from sweat, as well as subtle visible signals like blushing, pore and pupil dilation/constriction, and subtle audible frequencies like digestive fluctuations and a rumbling stomach. While we will explore an interplay of communication and internal physiological processes in later chapters, the primary focus of this book is on the use of vocal, facial, and bodily mechanisms used in forms of communication known as telereception.

DIRECT CONTACT COMMUNICATION VERSUS TELERECEPTION

According to Stefan Brudzynski, communication based on direct contact, whether mechanical or chemical, is phylogenetically older—meaning that it appeared much earlier in evolution than communication based on telereception. Telereception is anything sent across distance (tele meaning "far"). On earth, most of that will occur across air and water. In terms of telereception, there are two types that appear early in evolution: electroreception and distant chemoreception, or pheromones. Electroreception is the ability to detect electrostatic fields and is used predominantly by teleosts, a group of ray-finned fishes. Elasmobranchs, such as sharks and rays, and monotremes, egg-laying mammals like euchinids, as well as bumblebees [HOPKINS2017][1]. Visual and vocal communication appeared later in evolution, with mammals displaying the highest level of vocal sophistication [BRUDZYNSKI2010]. Visual and vocal communication in humans primarily involves the face, ears, voice, and body, all of which are under the influence of the somatic or voluntary nervous system. We are sending both voluntary and involuntary signals during our communicative interactions with others.

VOLUNTARY VERSUS INVOLUNTARY SYSTEMS

Using other humans in our social matrix is part of our survival and energy optimization process. To recruit humans into this process, we use various forms of communication, including audible, thermal, chemical, and visible signals. However, signals that occur due to changes in our autonomic systems are ones that are not under our voluntary control. These types of signals include pore and pupil dilation/constriction, smell, skin conductance, and temperature changes and occur in relation to fluctuations occurring within the autonomic nervous system. In contrast, the audible and visible signals we create using skeletal muscles are part of our somatic nervous system, which is under voluntary control. Within this system, muscles are attached to bones via tendons, communicate with nerves and blood vessels, and produce movement in

---

[1] In general, terrestrial animals do not have much use for electroreception: air has a high resistance that restricts the flow of electric current. However, humans are still able to detect strong electric currents (such as from batteries or static generators) via sensory-motor nerve fibers when they are in direct contact with an electric source or a conducting medium such as water. [HOPKINS2017]

all parts of the body. These muscles are striated, or striped, due to the various connective tissues that bind them together [BRITANNICADEC2022]. The movements that occur from these striated muscles' interactions with bones are voluntary. In contrast, pupil dilation, hair follicle changes (from goose-bumps, for example), pore dilations, and other actions are controlled by smooth muscles. Smooth muscles are tubular and not striped, contract slowly and automatically (not under voluntary control), and make up much of the musculature of the internal organs and digestive system as part of the auto-nomic nervous system [BRITANNICAFEB2022]. Both the somatic and autonomic systems are interrelated.

To illustrate the difference between these two systems, try the following:

- Look up and then down.
- Use your vocal muscles to hum.
- Raise your eyebrows.
- Clench your jaw.

All of these actions were part of your somatic nervous system. You used skel-etal muscles to move bones that created a visible or audible signal that some-one else could perceive with their eyes or ears.

Now try the following:

- Dilate your pupils.
- Contract the follicles of your hair to make goosebumps.
- Increase the conductance of your skin.
- Stop your intestinal tract from contracting.

As you likely observed, the above actions were not something you could acti-vate on command. The only way to trigger those changes would be to expose yourself to an environmental condition that would involuntarily trigger them. These actions are part of your autonomic nervous system. They are directed by smooth muscles, which are not under your voluntary control.

This is an important distinction because we do need to be aware that many of the signals, we transmit due to autonomic fluctuations that are beyond our awareness. They are indicators of our internal state. Although we cannot know what our pupils or skin conductance is doing at any given moment, we do have the ability to get better at knowing what our internal state is [CRAIG2002].

We can do this thanks to the sensations that occur within our internal organs that are sent up through the spinal cord and into the brain via afferent, also called "sensory," fibers. The awareness of our internal state through visceral sensations is called interoception [CAMERON2001]. Interoception is an important aspect of self-regulation because it acts as a form of internal feedback, which we explored in Chapter 2. In an upcoming section, we will see how internal feedback intertwines with the audible and visible signals we transmit and perceive via facial expressions and voice when we look at the component process model of emotion.

Eyes, Voice, and Face

In this section, we will keep our focus on how we create communication signals using mechanisms that are under our voluntary control, as well as how various signals that are not under our voluntary control can send signals to others that may affect behavior and communication patterns within dyads and groups. The focus in this section will be on eyes, voice, and facial expressions.

THE ROLE OF EYES IN COMMUNICATION

By 2 to 3 months of age, a pair of circles on a balloon representing a full face can induce an infant's smile, while a turning of the head to present only the side of the face and eliminating a representation of eyes can extinguish an infant's smile [SPITZ1965; COHN1987]. If a balloon with circles can elicit a smile in an infant, this says a lot about our eyes and the effect they have on other people's responses. Interestingly, research on face scanning shows that infants are most sensitive to facial affective expressions, in which specifically the eyes vary the most [HAITH1979].

There are three aspects of eyes that can influence the state of another:

- Pupil dilation
- Eye gaze
- Shape of eyes related to eyelids and muscles around the eyes

Pupil Dilation

As mentioned earlier, pupil dilation is controlled by smooth muscles and is, therefore, not under our voluntary control. Although we cannot control it, it is nevertheless helpful for our own understanding of communication to know that we are unconsciously affected by this signal in others. Pupillary dilation is an indicator of brain activity that is regulated by sympathetic networks in the hypothalamus, which is in contrast to the constriction of pupils mediated by the parasympathetic networks [TRUEX1964]. Pupillary changes are a reflection of internal states and brain activity. Some researchers assert that from an embryologic and anatomical perspective, the eye is in fact an extension of the brain [HESS1965]. Elevated sympathetic activity, which correlates with dilation of pupils, is also linked with a positive hedonic state in infants [LIPSITT1976]. Pupil dilation can create up to a fivefold change in the amount of light reaching the retina, which makes it an important feature for increasing the amount of information that can be perceived in a moment [GANONG1973]. In doing so, we can improve the snapshot we take of a person's emotional expressions and therefore more accurately sense their internal state and intentions. In one developmental study, infants smiled more when an experimenter's eyes were dilated versus constricted and large pupils in the infant elicited caregiver behavior [SCHORE1994].

Eye Gaze

Development researchers note that the most intense form of interpersonal communication from a neurological perspective is mediated by sustained facial gazing [TOMKINS1963; SCHORE2016]. In conjunction with pupil dilation, eye gaze also has biobehavioral effects on responses and communication patterns. Eye gaze and movements are controlled by muscles that originate in the eye socket (orbit) and work to move the eye up, down, side to side, and rotate the eye, with an additional muscle responsible for upper eyelid movement [DAVSON2023]. These extraocular muscles are under voluntary control [DAVSON2023]. Remember that voluntary control does not necessarily mean that we are *aware* of what we are doing with our eye gaze. Voluntary control means that we *can* deliberately adjust or inhibit movements using our skeletal muscles. Many of these movements, however, are happening so quickly and frequently that we are not paying attention to them. The fact that they are controlled by skeletal muscles, however, means that we can use our attentional focus and intention to move our eyes in one direction versus another. The way we move our eyes within interactions with others (which, to repeat, is generally happening without our conscious awareness) makes up our gaze patterns. Gaze patterns serve as visible signals for others to perceive our internal state and can trigger physiological arousal. These changes are reflected in electroencephalography (EEG) patterns, which are measurements in brainwave activity [GALE1972]. In fact, simply being the focus of attention of a member of the same species (a conspecific) can actually elevate physiological sensitivity to changes in the environment [CACIOPPO1990].

Extensive research shows that eye-to-eye contact gives advance notice of the intentions of a person, and the temporal structure of gaze provides clues to the readiness or capacity to receive and produce social information [RIESS1978]. When the eye gaze is fixated on an object or person and is coupled with eyebrows pulled down, and eyes widened and rounded, this can indicate interest-excitement [TOMKINS1963; IZARD1971]. Our noticing of someone's eye gaze can therefore serve as an indicator of their internal state and interest—in us or in an object or person they are tracking. As we saw in the previous chapter, eye gaze is also known to be a significant regulator of arousal states in infant-caregiver interactions [BRAZELTON1974; STERN1974]. Mutual eye contact in humans begins in approximately the infant's 4th week of life, with a dramatic increase in face fixations between 5 and 7 weeks [HAITH1977]. Developmental studies have shown that sustained levels of foveal (as opposed to peripheral) visual attention between caregiver and infant can lead to a crescendo in positive affect, as indicated by an infant's full-gape smile [BEEBE1977]. Other studies show that extended periods of maternal gaze elicit hormonal changes such as increases in endogenous opioids, enkephalins, and endorphins [HERMAN1978]. Interestingly, when mothers' behavior imitates the child, infant eye gaze increases, which researchers attribute to lower information processing demands for the infant and greater attentiveness and contingent responsiveness of the mother [FIELD1977].

THE ROLE OF FACIAL EXPRESSIONS IN COMMUNICATION

The visual perception of facial expressions has been shown in research to be the most salient form of nonverbal communication [IZARD1971]. Several challenges exist in the realm of studying facial expressions, however, and how they influence communication. Although facial expression has been the subjet of many years of research, the actual *mechanisms* of facial expression have received less focus [SCHERER2013]. As Scherer and colleagues suggest, this may be due to the fact that the majority of research has used static expressions such as in photos—which neglect the dynamic nature of facial movement used in communication. Moreover, emotion recognition has been the main focus of research, rather than the production of facial expressions. The challenge with this has been the assumption that there are prototypical facial muscle configurations that can be captured in a photograph and that these represent a small number of discrete emotions [SCHERER2019].

Various streams of research reflect different approaches to understanding emotion. Each theory highlights a specific idea that differentiates the theory from others. For example:

- Discrete emotion theory highlights the idea that emotion will produce a prototypical response and an emotion-specific pattern of facial expression [EKMAN1992; EKMAN1969; IZARD1994].

- Componential appraisal theory highlights the importance of appraisal as determining facial expression and motor behavior [SCHERER2009; SMITH1989; SMITH1997].

- Other researchers highlight the idea that facial expressions reflect the action readiness of an emotion [FRIJDA1997].

To help us understand how facial expressions are produced and perceived, a more comprehensive mechanical framework is helpful. One of these frameworks is the Tripartite Emotion Expression and Perception model (TEEP), [SCHERER2013]. This dynamic model is based on various frameworks proposed by Brunswik and Scherer's Component Process Model (CPM) of emotion [SCHERER2009; SCHERER2009A; BRUNSWIK1952]. These frameworks propose a dynamic, emergent unfolding of emotion processes that result in "symptoms" or externalizations, which are reflected in sequences of sign vehicles, including muscular movements in the face [SCHERER2013]. The observer then perceives these sign vehicles and appraises the significance of the expression using inference and attribution processes [SCHERER2013].

The Component Process Model of Emotion (CPM)

Because of its emphasis on the mechanical and physiological aspects of emotion expression, the CPM is a useful platform for exploring the biomechanics of how various nonverbal cues influence communication and behavior within human dynamics [SCHERER1984, 2001, 2009]. The CPM defines emotion as a process that occurs in reaction to salient events in the environment and reflects:

- Cognitive activity
- Physiological arousal

- Action tendencies

- Motor expression

- Subjective feeling state

Componential models of emotion suggest that different muscular elements that emerge in expressive facial configurations are driven by appraisals of an event, which are influenced by autonomic and somatic factors [SCHERER2013]. Specific response patterns that are observed during emotional scenes are unique, context-, and individual-specific. These patterns reflect a cumulated appraisal of stimuli based on the following [SCHERER2013]:

- Relevance of the event.

- How the event intersects with needs, goals, and values.

- The individual's ability to cope with the event and its consequences.

The relevance of the signals being appraised include a variety of factors, such as novelty or unexpectedness, pleasantness, or unpleasantness, and whether the event is perceived as being conducive or obstructive to satisfying a need, reach a goal, or uphold a value [SCHERER2001; ELLSWORTH2003]. A few key patterns stand out in terms of facial muscle movements as reflected in CPM research. To help understand these patterns, a review of some facial muscles may be useful.

Corrugator supercilii (brow region). This muscle is reflected in research as being related to frowning [YU2022].

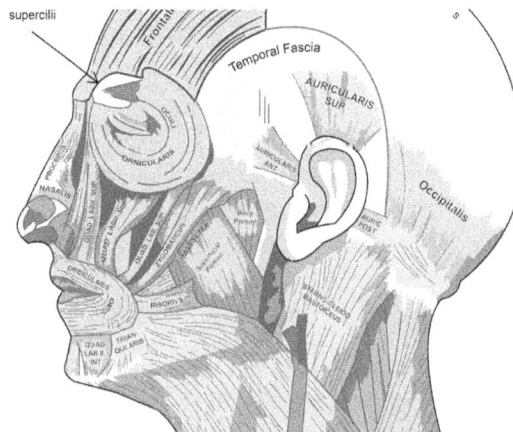

FIGURE 5.1 Corrugator Supercilii.

The **zygomaticus major muscle** (cheek region). This is a muscle that extends from each zygomatic arch (cheekbone) to the corners of the mouth. It is a muscle of facial expression that draws the angle of the mouth superiorly and posteriorly to allow one to smile [SCHMIDT2006].

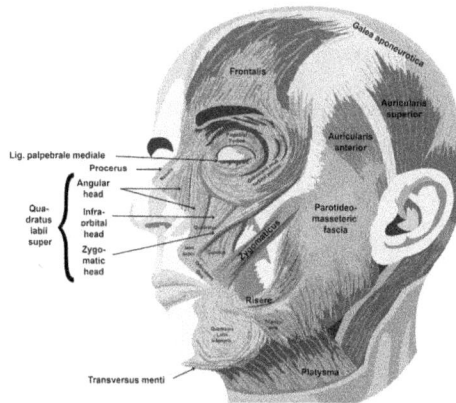

FIGURE 5.2 Zygomaticus Major.

Frontalis (forehead region). We see this region involved in eyebrow-raising [CHEN2015].

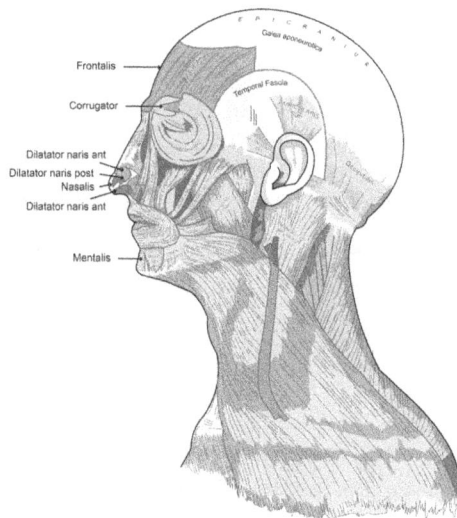

FIGURE 5.3 Frontalis.

The Frontalis is noted as the only muscle that raises the eyebrows and plays a major role in conveying emotions [CHEN2015].

As we look at various patterns of emotion expression, it is important to note that although the componential models of emotions attempt to make predictions about how an internal state manifests as observable configurations, these predictions are more probabilistic than deterministic [SCHERER2013]. Moreover, the link between appraisal and facial expression is difficult because:

- We can only have indirect access to how appraisals are occurring in an individual during emotional episodes.

- Most of the observations being studied occur in public or private settings where it can be difficult to record the face close-up.

- In public settings, there can be a tendency to suppress, modify, or mask emotions.

Some patterns in facial muscle configurations that have emerged from componential emotion research show increases in activation of the following facial muscle regions:

- Zygomaticus major (cheek region): noted for pleasant stimuli and goal-conducive events, smiling [SCHERER2013].

- Corrugator Supercilii (Brow region): unpleasant stimuli and goal-obstructive events. The corrugator in the brow region is linked with frowning. Appraisal of perceived obstacles was particularly responsible for frown activity [SCHERER2013].

- Frontalis (muscles over the forehead): Novel stimuli, eyebrow raise [CHEN2015; SCHERER2013].

- Forehead and brow region: unpleasant stimuli [SCHERER2013].

Although only probabilistic and not deterministic, evidence from the Component Processing Model supports predictions for three particular categories of appraisal [SCHERER2013]:

a) Appraisal of novelty: activity in the forehead (eyebrow raise) and eyelid opening.

b) Appraisal of intrinsic pleasantness: zygomaticus major, cheek raise (pleasant events), and corrugator (unpleasant events).

c) Appraisal of goal-related events: goal-conducive (zygomaticus major); goal-obstructive (corrugator).

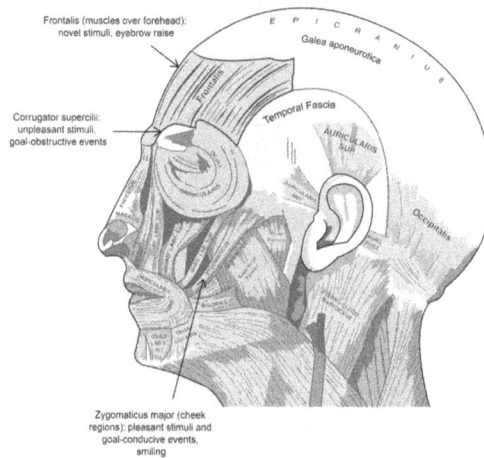

Frontalis (muscles over forehead): novel stimuli, eyebrow raise

Corrugator supercili: unpleasant stimuli, goal-obstructive events

Zygomaticus major (cheek regions): pleasant stimuli and goal-conducive events, smiling

FIGURE 5.4

EMBODIED COGNITION AND EMOTION EXPRESSION

An important innovation in our understanding of how learning and perception occur is the embodied cognition model [NIEDENTHAL2005; BARSALOU1999, 2008]. According to this model, learning and knowledge occur through sensorimotor simulations rather than abstract concepts. Barsalou's (1999) perceptual symbols systems (PSS) was one of the major influences of embodied cognition theory and proposed that thinking about an action triggers the same perceptual and sensory systems (e.g., auditory, visual, motor, and tactile) that occur during the act itself [BARSALOU2003, 2008]. This means that when we see and think about drinking from a bottle of water, for example, our brain activates various sensorimotor networks that simulate the movement of our hand grabbing the bottle, the feel of the liquid, the muscular fluctuations that occur as we hold the bottle in different angles [MACRINE2022]. The embodied cognition model has also been extended into emotion perception research, particularly for facial expressions. For example, one study using facial electromyography (EMG) found that participants simulated to some degree bodily components of anger and happiness when they interpreted faces with these concepts [HALBERSTADT2009]. When participants used "happy" to interpret an ambiguous expression, their own facial muscles simulated happiness: the zygomaticus activity was significantly stronger, and the corrugator activity weaker than when they encoded the face as "angry." When participants viewed nonemotion-related stimuli, there were no systematic changes in their own facial expressions [HALBERSTADT2009].

THE EFFECTS OF TRAUMA ON EMOTIONAL FACIAL EXPRESSION

The idea that our facial muscle movement influences and/or reflects how we experience emotional facial expressions is also reflected in research on patients with posttraumatic stress. Interestingly, in one study, traumatized female patients displayed equal amounts of facial expression as the control group but reported more arousal [WAGNER2003]. Moreover, the *less* they expressed facially, the more negative they reported feeling [WAGNER2003]. Less flexibility of expression can lead to poorer regulatory strategies and the ability to rebound after experiencing a stressful stimulus [WAGNER2003]. Acute traumatized patients have also been found to have a highly significant reduction of overall facial expression [KIRSCH2004]. Veterans show a special muscle activation pattern when viewing unpleasant combat-related material, which further suggests the important role facial emotional expression plays in posttraumatic stress [CARLSON1997].

Research on facial expressions during psychodynamic interviews revealed different patterns of facial behavior among traumatized patients compared with healthy controls, particularly when it came to enjoyment, anger, and contempt [KIRSCH2007]. In this study, the Emotional Facial Action Coding System (EMFACS) [FRIESEN1984; EKMAN2002] was used to register and analyze facial actions. The EMFACS is used to translate coded facial muscle movements into facial expressions of anger, contempt, disgust, fear, sadness, surprise, and enjoyment (which is reflected in a smile accompanied by wrinkles around the eyes, also known as the Duchenne smile[2]), and social smile (no wrinkles around the eyes) [FRIESEN1984; EKMAN2002]. Some important findings from this study include:

- The control group showed significantly more Duchenne smiles than the traumatized patients.

- Both groups (control group and patient group) showed similar patterns of eye gazing behavior; however, during mutual eye gaze, traumatized

---

[2] Duchenne smile: The Duchenne smile plays a powerful role in human interactions, and studies have found humans to be incredibly accurate when it comes to detecting the difference between inauthentic or social smiles compared with the Duchenne smile of authentic enjoyment [CITE__]

patients showed a reduction in Duchenne smiles, and the control group showed a significantly higher frequency of Duchenne smiles than the traumatized patients.

- Traumatized patients showed more negative effects, including anger, when eye contact was made (compared with the control group).

- The more contempt the traumatized patients showed, the more they attributed disgust to their interview.

- The more the traumatized patients expressed sadness, the more they had the impression that the interviewer experienced contempt.

The last two findings reveal a congruent coherence, which means that the patients had the impression that their negative emotions had a negative effect on the interviewer, and they attributed their own negative emotions to the interviewer [KIRSCH2007]. The findings of this study and similar studies have profound implications for what occurs during human communication and interaction. Here, we find that experiencing posttraumatic stress symptoms (in these studies, to a degree significant enough to be diagnosed with PTSD) reveals how intrusive trauma is: it affects a person's emotional experience and expression. If we think about, for example, parents and caregivers who are challenged with past trauma, we can see how much this can impact what occurs during interactions with their children and partners. For example, if eye gaze relates to facial configurations that reveal less enjoyment or even anger or contempt—these signals are being transmitted to the child or family member. As we saw in other studies, an aspect of how we learn is through sensorimotor simulation. If a child is attempting to engage in mutual eye gaze (which, as previously mentioned, is a developmental mechanism involved in regulating the nervous system as well as social referencing) and is met with lack of facial muscle movement around the eyes, or activation of the corrugator (anger), this activates a similar sensorimotor pattern in the child. The result will be a lack of soothing or regulating behavior.

As mentioned in Chapter 2, these nonverbal patterns are also used to create the internal working models used for future interactions. We can see some of this process reflected in studies that look at how nonverbal patterns may become translated into activation patterns. For example, people who had traumatic experiences during political imprisonment in the former German Democratic Republic have been noted as reporting more frequently on anger, which is reflected in a nonverbal pattern characterized by the propositional structure "the object has to go away" and a general "readiness to fight" [MAERCKER200]. In healthy dyads, this type of unconscious "go away!" effect based on past experiences does not occur; normal interactions generally include some form of "masking," "social smile," or "genuine joy"—all of which contribute to a type of social regulation pattern [KIRSCH2007]. Traumatized patients, on the other hand, have been found to lack this type of regulation pattern: the traumatic experience "breaks through," and the patients extend their negative experience to the interviewer [KIRSCH2007]. When we consider how many people may be affected by previous trauma—including many previous and current generations affected by war—we may begin to understand how much our social interactions could be influenced by the past. Understanding this can possibly lead us in new directions in terms of tools and frameworks for regulating ourselves when interacting with others (who may be transmitting social signals that are potentially more negative or lacking positive emotion-related patterns) as well as in ourselves and the signals we may be unconsciously transmitting to others.

SUMMARY

Not only do facial expressions reveal vast amounts of information pertaining to a person's internal experience and intentions, but the human voice is also another key player in social communication. Voice, facial expressions, and eyes all play a role in displaying our internal state as well as influencing the dynamics of communication and human interaction. The research presented in this chapter shows us how many different mechanisms interact to create signals that affect how our messages are transmitted to and received by others in powerful and often unconscious, ways. Various configurations of facial muscles and eye movements have direct effects on how people are perceived within social dynamics and can also indicate mental health challenges. The voluntary nature of these muscles being used to convey emotional and behavioral expressions means that we can become more aware and deliberate with how we use these muscles. Understanding this can be helpful in exploring therapeutic models, as well as deepening our understanding of how social dynamics can be assessed and addressed from a physically measurable and observable perspective of micro-movements. In the next chapter, we will continue this exploration of signal transmission and reception from a mechanical perspective of vocal and auditory systems.

REFERENCES

[BARSALOU1999]. Barsalou, L. W. (1999). Perceptual Symbol Systems. *Behavioral and Brain Sciences 1999, (22)*, 577–609.

[BARSALOU2003] Barsalou, L. W. (2003). Situated simulation in the human conceptual system. *Language and Cognitive Processes, 18*(5–6), 513–562.

[BARSALOU2008] Barsalou, L. W. (2002). Grounded cognition. *The Annual Review of Psychology (59)*, 617–645.

[BAYLISS2006] Bayliss, A. P., and Tipper, S. P. (2006). Predictive gaze cues and personality judgments: should eye trust you? *Psychological Science* 17, 514–520.

[BRITANNICADEC2022] Britannica, The Editors of Encyclopaedia. "skeletal muscle". *Encyclopedia Britannica*, 19 December 2022, *https://www.britannica.com/science/skeletal-muscle*. Accessed 29 December 2022.

[BRITANNICAFEB2022] Britannica, The Editors of Encyclopaedia. "smooth muscle". *Encyclopedia Britannica*, 6 February 2022, *https://www.britannica.com/science/smooth-muscle*. Accessed 29 December 2022.

[BRUNSWIK1952] Brunswick, E. (1952). *The Conceptual Framework of Psychology*. Chicago: Chicago University Press.

[BURGOON2021] Burgoon, J. K., Wang, X., Chen, X., Pentland, S. J., and Dunbar, N. E. (2021). Nonverbal behaviors "speak" relational messages of dominance, trust, and composure. *Frontiers in Psychology (12)*, 624177.

[CARLSON1997] Carlson, J. G., Singelis, T. M., and Chemtob, C.M. (1997). Facial EMG responses to combat-related visual stimuli in veterans with and without posttraumatic stress disorder. *Applied Psychophysiology and Biofeedback, (22)*, 247–259.

[CHEN2015] Chen, Y., Yang, Z., and Wang, J. (2015). Eyebrow emotional expression recognition using surface EMG signals. *Neurocomputing (168)*, 871–879.

[COHN1987] Cohn, J. F., and Tronick, E. Z. (1987). Mother-infant face-to-face interaction: the sequence of dyadic states at 3, 6, and 9 months. *Developmental Psychology (23)*, 1, 68–77.

[COLLIN2019] Collin, S. P. (2019). *Encyclopedia of Animal Behavior* (second edition). San Diego: Academic Press.

[DAVSON2023] Davson, H.., and Perkins, E. S. "Human eye". *Encyclopedia Britannica*, 19 April 2023, *https://www.britannica.com/science/human-eye*. Accessed 1 July 2023.

[EKMAN1992] Ekman, P. (1992). Facial expressions of emotion: New findings, new questions. *Psychological Science, 3*, 34–38.

[EKMAN1969] Ekman, P., Sorenson, E. R., and Friesen, W. V. (1969). Pancultural elements in facial displays of emotion. *Science, 164*, 86–88.

[ELLIS1989]. Ellis, A.W. (1989). Neuro-cognitive processing of faces and voices. In H.D. Young and A. W. Ellis (Eds.), *Handbook of Research on Face Processing* (pp. 207–215). Amsterdam, The Netherlands: Elsevier Science Publications B.V.

[ELLSWORTH2002] Ellsworth, P. C., and Scherer, K. R. (2003). Appraisal processes in emotion. In *Handbook of Affective Sciences* (pp. 572–595), Davidson, R., Scherer, K. R., and Goldsmith, H. H. (eds.). New York, NY: Oxford University Press.

[FIELD1977]. Field, T. M. (1977). Effects of early separation, interactive deficits, and experimental manipulations on infant-mother face-to-face interaction. *Child Development, 3* (48), 763–771.

[FRANCE2000] France, D. J., Shiavi, R. G., Silverman, M., and Wilkes, M. (2000). Acoustical properties of speech as indicators of depression and suicidal risk. *IEEE Transactions on Biomedical Engineering, 47*, 829–837.

[FRIJDA1997] Frijda, N. H., and Tcherkassof, A. (1997). Facial expressions as modes of action readiness. In *The psychology of facial expression* (pp. 78–102), J. A. Russell and J. M. Fernández-Dols (eds.). Cambridge, UK: Cambridge University Press.

[HAITH1977] Haith, M. M., Bergman, T., and Moore, M. J. (1977). Eye contact and face scanning in early infancy. *Science, 198*(4319), 853–855.

[HAITH1979] Haith, M. M., Bergman, T., and Moore, M. (1979). Eye contact and face scanning in early infancy. *Science, 218*, 179–181.

[HERMAN1978] Herman, B. H., aand Panskepp, J. (1978). Evidence for opiate mediation of social affect. *Pharmacological Biochemistry and Behavior, 9*, 213–220.

[HESS1965] Hess, E. H. (1965) Attitude and pupil size. *Scientific American, 212*, 46–54.

[IZARD1971] Izard, C.E. (1971). *The Face of Emotion.* New York: Appleton-Century-Crofts.

[IZARD1994] Izard, C. E. (1994). Innate and universal facial expressions: Evidence from developmental and cross-cultural research. *Psychological Bulletin, 115*, 288–299.

[JUSLIN2001] Juslin, P. N., and Laukka, P. (2001). Impact of intended emotion intensity on cue utilization and decoding accuracy in vocal expression of emotion. *Emotion (Washington, D.C.), 1*, 381–412.

[KIRSCH2005] Kirsch, A., and Brunnhuber, S. (2007). Facial expression and experience of emotions in psychodynamic interviews with patients with PTSD in comparison to healthy subjects. *Psychopathology, 40*, 296–302.

[KRUMHUBER2007] Krumhuber, E., Manstead, A. S., Cosker, D., Marshall, D., Rosin, P. L., and Kappas, A. (2007). Facial dynamics as indicators of trustworthiness and cooperative behavior. *Emotion, 7*, 730–735.

[MACRINE2022] Macrine, S. L., and Fuguate, J. M. B. (eds.) (2022). *Movement Matters: How Embodied Cognition Informs Teaching and Learning.* Cambridge, MA: The MIT Press. 10.7551/mitpress/13593.001.0001

[MOORE2003] Moore, E., Clements, M. Peifer, J., & Weisser, L. (2003, September 17–21). Analysis of prosodic variation in speech for clinical depression. In *Proceedings of the 25th Annual International Conference of the IEEE Engineering in Medicine and Biology Society* (Vol. 3, pp. 2925–2928), IEEE (Ed.). Cancun, Mexico.

[NEGUS1949] Negus, V. E. (1949). *The Comparative Anatomy and Physiology of the Larynx.* London: W. Heinemann Medical Books.

[NIEDENTHAL2005] Niedenthal, P. M., Barsalou, L. W., Winkielman, P., KrauthGruber, S., and Ric, F. (2005). Embodiment in attitudes, social perception, and emotion. *Personality and Social Psychology Review, 9*, 184–211.

[PESSINO2022] Pessino, K., Patel, J., and Patel, B. C. (2022). *Anatomy, Head and Neck, Frontalis Muscle.* StatPearls Publishing: Treasure Island, FL.

[PITTAM1993] Pittam, J., and Scherer, K. R. (1993). Vocal expression and communication of emotion. In *Handbook of emotions* (pp. 185–198), Lewis, M., and Haviland, J. M. (eds.). New York: Guilford Press.

[POLLERMANN2002]. Pollerman, B. Z., and Archinard, M. (2002). Acoustic patterns of emotions. In *Improvements in Speech Synthesis* (pp. 237–245), Keller, E., Bailly, G., Monaghan, A., Terken, J., and Huckvale, M. (eds.). Chichester, England: John Wiley & Sons.

[RIESS1978] Riess, A. (1978). The mother's eye: for better and for worse. *Psychoanalytic Study of the Child, 33*, 381–409.

[SANVICTORES2022] Sanvictores, T., and Tadi, P. Neuroanatomy, autonomic nervous system visceral afferent fibers and pain. [Updated 2022 Oct 3]. In: StatPearls [Internet]. Treasure Island (FL): StatPearls Publishing; 2022 January.

[SCHERER1979] Scherer, K.R. (1979). Nonlinguistic Vocal Indicators of Emotion and Psychopathology. In: Izard, C.E. (eds) Emotions in Personality and Psychopathology. Emotions, Personality, and Psychotherapy. Springer, Boston, MA. *https://doi.org/10.1007/978-1-4613-2892-6_18*

[SCHERER1986] Scherer, K. R. (1986). Vocal affect expression: a review and a model for future research. *Psychological Bulletin, 99*, 143–165.

[SCHERER2001] Scherer, K. R. (2001). Appraisal considered as a process of multilevel sequential checking. In *Appraisal Processes in Emotion: Theory, Methods, Research* (pp. 92–120), Scherer, K. R., Schorr, A., and Johnstone, T. (eds.). New York, NY: Oxford University Press.

[SCHERER2009] Scherer, K. R. (2009). The dynamic architecture of emotion: Evidence for the component process model. *Cognition & Emotion, 23*, 1307–1351.

[SCHERER2009A] Scherer, K. R. (2009). Emotions are emergent processes: they require a dynamic computational architecture. *Philosophical Transactions of the Royal Society of London. Series B, Biological Sciences, 364*(1535), 3459–3474.

[SCHERER2011] Scherer, K. R., Clark-Polner, E., and Mortillaro, M. (2011). In the eye of the beholder? Universality and cultural specificity in the expression and perception of emotion, *International Journal of Psychology, 46*(6), 401–435.

[SCHERER2013] Scherer, K. R., Mortillaro, M., and Mehu, M. (2013). Understanding the mechanisms underlying the production of facial expression of emotion: a componential perspective. *Emotion Review, 5*, 47–53. doi: 10.1177/1754073912451504

[SCHERER2019] Scherer, K. R. (2019) Dynamic facial expression of emotion and observer inference. *Frontiers in Psychology, 10,* 508

[SCHMIDT2006] Schmidt, K. L., Ambadar, Z., Cohn, J. F., et al. (2006). Movement differences between deliberate and spontaneous facial expressions: *Zygomaticus Major* action in smiling. *The Journal of Nonverbal Behavior, 30,* 37–52.

[SCHON1995] Schön Ybarra, M. (1995). A comparative approach to the non-human primate vocal tract: Implications for sound production. In *Frontiers in Primate Vocal Communication* (pp. 185–198), Zimmerman, E., and Newman, J. D. (eds.). Boston: Plenum Press.

[SCHORE1994] Schore, A. (1994) *Affect Regulation and the Origin of the Self: The Neurobiology of Emotional Development.* Hillsdale, NJ: Erlbaum.

[SMITH1989] Smith, C. A. (1989). Dimensions of appraisal and physiological response in emotion. *Journal of Personality and Social Psychology, 56,* 339–353.

[SMITH1997] Smith, C. A., and Scott, H. (1997). A componential approach to the meaning of facial expressions. In *The psychology of facial expression* (pp. 229–254), J. A. Russell & J. M. Fernández-Dols (eds.). New York, NY: Cambridge University Press.

[SPITZ1965] Spitz, R. (1965). *The first year of life.* New York: International Universities Press.

[TOMKINS1963] Tomkins, S. (1963). *Affect/Imagery/Consciousness: Vol. 2. The Negative Affects.* New York: Springer.

[VOGL2020] Vogl, E., Pekrun, R., Murayama, K., and Loderer, K. (2020). Surprised-curious-confused: Epistemic emotions and knowledge exploration. *Emotion, 20*(4), 625–641. doi: 10.1037/emo0000578.

[WAGNER2003] Wagner, A. W., Roemer, L. Orsillo, S. M., and Litz, B. T. (2003). Emotional experiencing in women with posttraumatic stress disorder: congruence between facial expressivity and self-report. *Journal of Traumatic Stress, 16,* 67–75.

[YU2022] Yu, M., and Wang, S. M. Anatomy, Head and Neck, Eye Corrugator Muscle. [Updated 2022 Aug 8]. In: StatPearls [Internet]. Treasure Island (FL): StatPearls Publishing; 2023 Jan-. Available from: *https://www.ncbi.nlm.nih.gov/books/NBK542280/*

6

COMMUNICATION AND THE VOICE-HEART CONNECTION

Read the following three items in your head or aloud with their corresponding punctuation: (1) "Hello!!!" (2) "Hello." (3) "Hello???" Did you notice a change in the tone or inflections of your voice as you read each word? If you read the words in your head, did you notice an internal voice and changes in tone or inflection? Our written words and punctuation are a reflection of what our voices do when we speak. For example, as you read a question, perhaps you notice that there is a certain pitch that changes at the end of the sentence, right before the question mark. Punctuation is a graphical method of emulating some of the vocal features we use to convey information about our internal state and intentions. Other ways we convey information come from how we use our breathing and vocal muscles to create different effects. For example, how someone's tone and loudness of voice may affect how you perceive the interaction. Do quieter, more melodic voices induce a different reaction in you than loud, abrupt, or barking voices? In Chapter 5, we looked at some of the mechanics of communication signals transmitted and received via facial configurations that are associated with internal states and evaluations of affect. In this chapter, we will look at how the voice and our auditory systems play a role in our communication signals and patterns. Voice has both verbal and nonverbal elements: we will begin our exploration with nonverbal vocalizations and the auditory system in this chapter, and in the following chapter, we will examine the formation and role of words and symbols within communication.

VOICE AND COMMUNICATION

Extensive research over decades has revealed that a large number of emotional and motivational states can be indexed and communicated using specific acoustic characteristics and configurations [BANSE1996]. More than a century ago, Helmholtz noted that voice plays a critical role in reflecting one's state of mind [VANDENBROEK2004]. The cumulation of past and current research on voice shows us that minute inter- and intra-individual variations of speech patterns carry useful information that helps us recognize a person's identity and emotions [BERLIN2004; ELLIS1989]. Different emotional and motivational states contain specific acoustic features that allow humans to recognize and differentiate between these states [BANSE1996]. Humans share information via vocalization, both verbally and nonverbally. Verbal vocalization consists of speech, which is a vocal form of symbolic representation of information (language). Within this verbal form of vocalization, information is transmitted through semantics (including linguistic phrases and lexical meanings)—this is related to "what" is being said [KAMILOGLU2021]. Speech prosody is the rhythmic and intonational aspect of speech and includes modulation of pitch, amplitude, and speech rate to communicate emotions in concurrence with semantic content—this is related to "how" something is being said [KAMILOGLU2021]. For example, a raise in pitch at the end of a sentence can indicate a question. Nonverbal vocalizations are brief nonspeech vocalizations also called "affect bursts" [SCHERER1994]. These can include sighs, laughs, and grunts and are potent carriers of emotional information that develop early in ontogeny [SCHERER1994]. We will deepen our exploration of how voice conveys emotions and internal states in upcoming sections of this chapter. Before going into that, we will take an initial look at some of the physiological mechanisms associated with vocal production, including how our respiration, heart rhythms, and internal state are intertwined with voice frequencies.

THE VOICE-FACE-HEART CONNECTION

You may have noticed that it seems easier to detect the motivational state of a dog than it is to detect this in a fish or turtle. While the speed and direction of body movements can give us some clues for a variety of species, there are other changes that happen in mammals that offer additional information. This information is found particularly in the sounds of vocalizations as well as facial configurations. The voice-face-heart connection is a mammalian system that integrates facial expressions, vocalizations, and neural regulation of autonomic systems, including heart rhythms and blood flow [PORGES2021]. This integrated system is what allows mammals to detect and transmit signals to one another to indicate if it is safe to approach or that one or both members of an interaction are in a reactive and mobilized state that could make an interaction dangerous [PORGES2021]. Various theories have emerged over time to explore this facet of social interaction that includes bidirectional communication between the brain and the heart as a basis for interactive regulation. Darwin suggested the influence of the vagus nerve on these systems, and other scientists have continued that exploration [LORENZA2017]. Claude Bernard's heart-brain connection theories and Thayer and Lane's Neurovisceral Integration Model have been influential in much of this field of research [THAYER2009]. In addition, the polyvagal theory, and its related social engagement system developed by Stephen Porges, emerged from studies on neonates and heart rhythms and further developed a theory involving the vagus nerve and various systems that regulate heart-brain communication, facial gestures, middle ear muscles, and vocal communication [LORENZA2017; PORGES2021; PORGES2001].

Voice output is part of a psychophysiological system that integrates sympathetic and parasympathetic mechanisms to help us respond to environmental opportunities and challenges [THAYER2009; VANPUYVELDE2018]. The rich amount of socially relevant information contained in vocalizations can influence many different aspects of behavior, from mate selection to how people are perceived in job interviews and political platforms [KLOFSTAD2015; PISANSKI2019]. Humans and other species can also increase their chance of survival by how accurately they perceive and respond to conspecific alarm calls when there is a nearby predator [ADOLPHS2018]. Vocalization involves a complex coordination of simultaneous increases and decreases, reciprocal, or independent responses from the sympathetic and parasympathetic nervous systems [BERNTSON1991]. Mammalian vocalization is a particularly important conveyor of internal state because of how heart rhythms, breathing and voice are related [DEMARTSEV2022]. Mammals, and not reptiles, are able to coordinate the effort and volume of respiration as a way to manipulate voice frequencies [PORGES2021]. This is possible due to two distinct but interrelated vagal circuits that exist in mammals: one that deals with the subdiaphragmatic organs and one that deals with supradiaphragmatic organs [PORGES2001; PORGES2021. The subdiaphragmatic branch of the vagus regulates abdominal breathing, and the supradiaphragmatic vagus coordinates laryngeal and pharyngeal muscles, and muscles involved in facial expressions [PORGES2021].

The mammalian—and human—ability to coordinate respiration with vocalizations allows us to not only convey information about the environment, but because it is tied to breathing, it also directly reflects our internal state. An example of this is in medically compromised human infants. Infant cries are regulated by neural tone via circuits in the nucleus ambiguus, which connect to the pharyngeal and laryngeal muscles and the heart [LESTER1982; PORTER1988]. Physiologically distressed infants produce high-pitched cries in short bursts that have little frequency modulation [LESTER1982; PORTER1988]. The dramatic increase in heart rate and respiration and the fundamental frequency of their cry during these distressed states suggest a decrease in cardiac vagal tone [PORGES2021]. Research on infant circumcision reflects this pain-voice-heart connection: newborn pain cries in response to circumcision are high-pitched and paralleled with significantly reduced cardiac vagal tone [PORTER1988]. This reduction in cardiac vagal tone is measured by respiratory sinus arrhythmia and is mediated via myelinated vagal pathways that originate in the nucleus ambiguous [PORGES2021]. Reduced cardiac vagal tone is an indication of sympathetic nervous system hyperarousal [LABORDE2017].

In other mammalian vocalizations, such as in rats, we also see this connection between internal state and the modulation of vocalizations. Adult rats have two types of vocalizations: one is audible to humans, or sonic, and has a fundamental frequency between 2 and 4 kHz with rich harmonic elements [NITSCHKE1982]. The other is ultrasonic, between 20 and 70 kHz and possibly as high as 100 kHz, and maybe used as a defensive threat vocalization [LITVIN2007]. Different frequencies are associated with different activities and situations: short 50 kHz ultrasonic vocalizations with varying degrees of frequency are associated with sexual and aggressive interactions, while longer 22 kHz vocalizations have been found to occur in a variety of other situations including submission, alarm, and post-copulatory periods [CONSTANINI2006; PORTFORS2007]. While playing and experiencing positive affective states, rats transmit ultrasonic vocalizations across a range of frequencies [BRUDZYNSKI2010]. While adult ultrasonic calls appear to be most related to aggression and mating, infant ultrasonic calls have the power to initiate parent retrieval and minimize rough parental handling [NYBY2010]. Adolescent rats emit ultrasonic calls in response to rough and tumble play as well as human tickling [PANSKEPP2000]. Primates, such as rhesus monkeys, also have nervous system fluctuations in response to species-specific threat calls and reflect activation of the sympathetic nervous system as measured by a decrease in skin temperature and induction of skin conductance response (SCR) in the upper nasal region [KURAOKA2010; BOUCSEIN1992; KISTLER1998]

HUMAN VOICE MECHANISMS AND FEATURES

The frequency, pitch, loudness, quality, and prosody of human voice conveys valuable information and is a fundamental aspect of human communication beyond words and gestures, which we will explore in Chapter 7. Human voice can convey various forms of information such as size, age, gender, as well as more transitory states such as health and power [KREIMAN2011]. Some vocalizations are not necessarily intended to affect the behavior of another and occur spontaneously due to physiological changes such as when tickled or in pain. These types of vocalizations are considered cues [WILEY1978]. In this section, we will focus specifically on vocalizations that serve as a form of behavioral transmitter and are intended to influence the behavior and state of another. Vocalizations that serve to influence behavior are considered communicative and are categorized as signals [WILEY1978]. A major aspect of communicative vocalization lies in its ability to transmit information about not just internal physiological state changes but also emotions. Scherer and colleagues' research has shown that human vocalizations conveying emotional states such as anger, fear, and sadness each carry their own unique acoustic profile [SCHERER1986].

Before we explore voice features associated with affect and emotions, it may be helpful to have an overview of voice production and common acoustic features of voice.

The Physiological Basis of Vocalizing

Vocal production consists of three main components [LIEBERMAN1988]:

- Subglottal system (includes the trachea and lungs)
- Larynx (contains the vocal folds)
- Supralaryngeal vocal tract (includes the nasal cavity, oral cavity, and pharynx)

The subglottal system generates airflow and consists of the lungs and trachea (a single tube that branches into two airways leading into a lung) [SUNDBERG2013]. As mammals, we can increase or decrease the volume of our lungs by contracting expiratory or inspiratory muscles. During inhalation, we use inspiratory muscles to expand the thoracic cavity. Muscles that induce exhalation by compressing the thoracic cavity are called expiratory muscles [LEVANGIE2011]. Exhaled air from the lungs drives the oscillations of the vocal folds (often called "vocal cords"). The air pressure from the lungs blows the vocal folds apart and sucks them together in a cyclical way [KAMILOGLU2021]. The rapid and repetitive movements of vocal folds are due to changes in subglottal air pressure and the elasticity of the glottis. These oscillations modulate the airflow and produce vocalization [ZHANG2016].

The sound produced by the rate of oscillation in the vocal folds is called the fundamental frequency of pitch, or *F0*. Generally, this pitch is about 100 Hz in adult men and about 200 Hz in adult women [VANDENBROEK2004]. As the acoustic energy from these oscillations passes through the supralaryngeal vocal tract (the pharynx, oral and nasal cavities), it is filtered and then finally moves through the nostrils and mouth into the environment [KAMILOGLU2021]. The shape and length of the supralaryngeal tract changes continuously during vocalization, which produces different sounds [KAMILOGLU2021]. The filtering process that occurs through the changes in the length and shape of the vocal tract plays a crucial role in speech and is reflected in the source-filter theory.

Source-filter theory

The source-filter theory illustrates vocalizations as a two-stage process: first, sound is produced from a source, and then filtered [FANT1960]. The subglottal system generates airflow—but this alone does not produce the sound. The *source* of sound is the transformation of airflow into vibrations via the vocal folds in the larynx [SUNDBERG2013]. The spectrum of sounds comes from the shaping and filtering that occurs in the vocal tract (the *filter*) [KAMILOGLU2021]. The length and shape of the vocal tract determine how sounds are emitted, allowing specific frequencies to pass unhindered, while blocking others. This series of "bandpass filters" are called formants. These formants are rapidly modulated during speech by the articulators (tongue, lips, soft palate, etc.) [VANDENBROECK2004].

The source-filter principle can be applied to virtually all vertebrate vocal productions, but there are some differences between humans and other primates when it comes to the position of larynx and the lack of air sacs in humans [FANT1960; KAMILOGLU2021]. Early in infancy, the larynx is lowered in the human vocal tract, which gives the tongue more space to move and increases articulatory flexibility [SCHON1995]. Humans also have a particularly long vocal tract, which enables them to create a wider variety of vocal tract shapes [LIEBERMAN1969]. The extra space for tongue movement and variety of vocal tract shapes allows humans to create a distinctly large range of variation in formant frequencies and enhanced vocal tract filtering to create even more distinct sounds [KAMILOGLU2021]. Some mammals such as lions and koalas are capable of dynamically lowering the larynx in the vocal tract [FITCH2000]. This suggests that a descended larynx is not the only aspect of the distinct variety of novel vocalizations produced by humans. Another anatomical difference is that humans do not have sac-like extensions of the larynx, while many nonhuman primates and other mammals do [FITCH2018; NEGUS1949]. Human anatomical developments related to speech and vocal production therefore include the lack of laryngeal air sacs and a permanently descended larynx. These combined with control over breathing and control of the tongue, vocal folds, and shape of the chin all contribute to the wide range of vocalizations in humans [DEBOER2019].

The source-filter theory is a key insight from modern speech research because it highlights how source and filter features can be controlled independently: the formants (determined by the vocal tract, aka *filter*) are independent of the fundamental frequency of pitch (determined by the vocal fold vibration rate, aka *source*) [KAMILOGLU2021]. The independent control of source and filter means that various features of voice, such as intensity, amplitude, and sound configurations, are formed by tensions and changes in different muscles and within different systems. These changes involve our breath and other mechanisms that can be influenced by our internal state and emotional arousal, thus influencing voice patterns and profiles. The source-filter theory is helpful in identifying these acoustic features for emotions because it allows researchers to connect acoustics with physiological state [SCHERER1986].

Emotions in the voice can be expressed through verbal aspects such as linguistic meaning and semantics (discussed in Chapter 7), as well as through nonverbal vocalizations and acoustic features. Some common acoustic features of vocalizations are as follows:

F_0 **(Fundamental Frequency) fundamental frequency** is produced by the rate of oscillation in the vocal folds. It is measured in Hertz (Hz), which is the number of cycles per second. The fundamental frequency is the lowest frequency of a periodic waveform[1] [KAMILOGLU2021]. Because it is the lowest frequency, it is often perceived as the loudest and is thus identified as a specific pitch [BENWARD1997/2003]. Fundamental frequency is therefore also sometimes called fundamental frequency of pitch, or *F0* [KAMILOGLU2021]. Pitch is the highness or lowness of a sound based on the rate of vibration. Something that is vibrating faster therefore produces a higher pitched sound than something vibrating at a lower rate. Frequencies are something that are objectively measurable, while pitch is the *perception* of the frequency [KAMILOGLU2021]. For pitch, the listener attributes a certain tone that is relative to other tones on a musical scale (so a pitch is higher or lower to others on this scale) [KAMILOGLU2021]. Generally, the fundamental frequency of pitch in humans is about 100 Hz in adult men and about 200 Hz in adult women [VANDENBROEK2004]. As the acoustic energy from these oscillations passes through the supralaryngeal vocal tract (the pharynx, oral, and nasal cavities), it is filtered and then finally moves through the nostrils and mouth into the environment. The shape and length of the supralaryngeal tract changes continuously during vocalization, and these changes produce different sounds [KAMILOGLU2021]. This filtering process that occurs through the changes in the length and shape of the vocal tract plays a crucial role in speech and is reflected in the source-filter theory.

F_1, F_2,... (Formant Frequencies): Formant frequencies, or formants, are peaks in the frequency spectrum that have a high degree of energy [KAMILOGLU2021]. For example, as someone speaks, they change the shape of the vocal tract, which then filters the sounds they express. This variable acoustic filter allows more energy at certain frequencies. These peaks in energy are the formants. They are especially prominent in vowels [ABHANG2016]. You may be able to detect a difference in the amount of energy coming from the sounds you make when you hear yourself saying vowel sounds such as "ah," "eh," "oh" versus consonants "f," "s," "p," "d," etc.

Amplitude: Amplitude is related to the air pressure in a wave and is therefore a measurement of the amount of energy that it carries [KAMILOGLU2021]. Amplitude affects the intensity: a sound with higher amplitude would be perceived as louder (higher intensity) than a sound with lower amplitude or energy [LUMEN2021; URONE2020].

---

[1] Periodic waveform: Periodic refers to an interval that repeats regularly. Waveform is the shape of the wave.

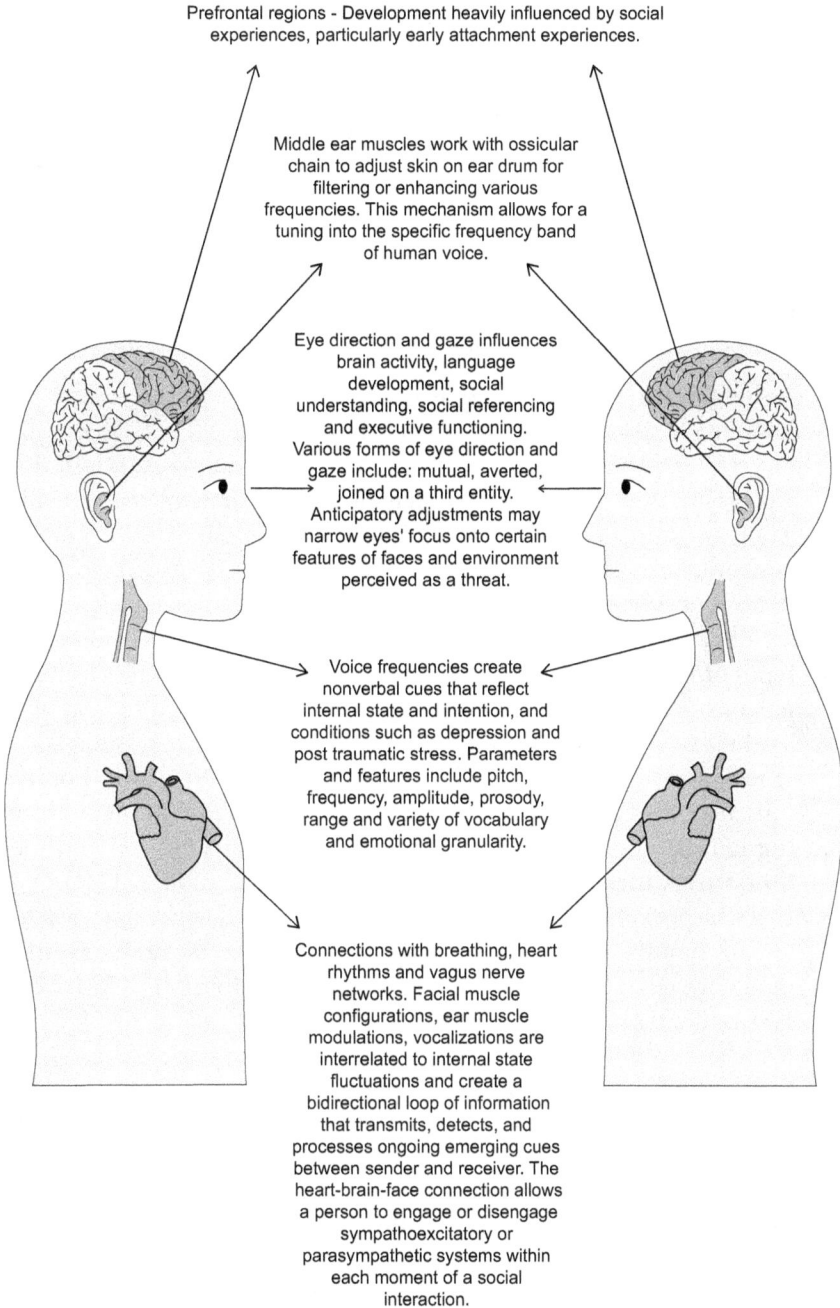

Prefrontal regions - Development heavily influenced by social experiences, particularly early attachment experiences.

Middle ear muscles work with ossicular chain to adjust skin on ear drum for filtering or enhancing various frequencies. This mechanism allows for a tuning into the specific frequency band of human voice.

Eye direction and gaze influences brain activity, language development, social understanding, social referencing and executive functioning. Various forms of eye direction and gaze include: mutual, averted, joined on a third entity. Anticipatory adjustments may narrow eyes' focus onto certain features of faces and environment perceived as a threat.

Voice frequencies create nonverbal cues that reflect internal state and intention, and conditions such as depression and post traumatic stress. Parameters and features include pitch, frequency, amplitude, prosody, range and variety of vocabulary and emotional granularity.

Connections with breathing, heart rhythms and vagus nerve networks. Facial muscle configurations, ear muscle modulations, vocalizations are interrelated to internal state fluctuations and create a bidirectional loop of information that transmits, detects, and processes ongoing emerging cues between sender and receiver. The heart-brain-face connection allows a person to engage or disengage sympathoexcitatory or parasympathetic systems within each moment of a social interaction.

FIGURE 6.1

Voice intensity: This is the energy through the unit area carried by a soundwave, such as square meters of air per second. A more intense sound will come from a source that can produce larger amplitude oscillations [LUMEN2021]. As the amplitude of the sound wave increases, voice intensity increases. This is perceived by a listener as *loudness* [KAMILOGLU2021]. Vocalizations with different fundamental frequencies (f0) and amplitudes are illustrated on this website: *https://emotionwaves.github.io/acoustics*

Speech rate: Speech rate refers to the number of vocalized elements (e.g., syllables or words) per time unit (such as seconds) [DEMENKO2012]. It can also be measured by how long it takes to say a word or other structure.

Voice Quality: Voice quality is the overall "coloring" of voice is the result of how much vibration occurs at each frequency [SCHERER1986]. Examples of voice qualities are modal, creaky, or whispering [KAMILOGLU2021], as well as hoarseness, breathiness, harshness, and creakiness [SCHERER1986]. These qualities convey important information about a person's emotional state and intentions [ANIKIN2020; GRICHKOVSTSOVA2012]. Voice qualities are determined by vocal fold configurations that change aerodynamic flow such as subglottal pressure and glottal air flow, and which are influenced by three types of muscular tension: adductive tension, medial compression, longitudinal tension [GOBL2010]. For example, the most frequent kind of voice quality during normal speech is modal voice and is produced when the vocal folds vibrate as a single unit [KAMILOGLU2021; ESLING2019]. For modal voice, muscular tension (adductive tension, medial compression, and longitudinal tension) is moderate. For creaky voice, adductive tension and medial compression are high, but there is little longitudinal tension [KAMILOGLU2021]. In a whispering voice, the hissing sound is created when the vocal folds do not vibrate but are separated by a gap, and involves low adductive tension, and moderate medial compression and longitudinal tension [KAMILOGLU2021; ESLING2019].

Other acoustic features of voice include jitter, shimmer, spectral energy, global waveform, harmonics-to-noise ratio (HNR) and prosody [CUMMINS2015].

Jitter and shimmer reflect perturbations and voice stability or instability. Jitter relates to the variations (perturbations) of fundamental frequency.

Shimmer relates to perturbations in amplitude. A normal voice naturally contains certain amounts of variability and instability in f0 and amplitude; however, large perturbations or inconsistencies can be captured by instruments and calculations that assess jitter and shimmer [CUMMINS2015].

Spectral energy is related to the proportion of high-frequency energy that is distributed within a vocalization [YINGTHAWORNSUK2007]. When the proportion of high-frequency energy increases, this results in a voice that sounds sharper and less soft.

Harmonic-to-Noise Ratio (HNR) is a measurement of the relationship between the periodic component (harmonic part) and aperiodic component (noise) of a voice and is expressed in decibels (dB)[FERNANDES2018]. This signal varies due to different vocal tract configurations that lead to different amplitudes and harmonics: a lower value indicates a noisier vocalization, while a higher level indicates a more tonal sound [FERNANDES2018].

Prosody refers to variations in perceived rhythm, stress, and intonation of speech, pitch, and loudness [CUMMINS2015].

Speech Production

Speech recruits various major muscle groups and involves more motor fibers than any other human mechanical activity [KENT2000]. Along with neuro-muscular commands, speech production also involves simultaneous cognitive planning and the need for short-term memory (working memory), analysis of visual information, and language comprehension [BADDELEY2003]. As we speak, we continuously monitor and adjust our vocalizations via an auditory feedback loop and proprioceptive feedback loop, which makes us aware of our muscles' movements [POSTMA2000].

Voice Features and Affective State

Acoustic features of voice can contain information about a person's affective state, which relates to physiological changes and arousal levels that include changes in the machinery used to produce voice [SCHERER1986]. The Component Patterning Theory proposes a model for predicting and analyzing vocal patterns of various affective states that are related to a multitude of components such as novelty, goal achievement, and perceived ability to cope. Some examples of these predictions include [SCHERER1986]:

- Sudden inhalation and interruption of phonation in response to novel stimuli.

- Low-to-moderate amplitude and decrease in high-frequency energy in response to stimuli that are relevant and consistent with goals.

▪ Deep forceful respiration and strong energy in the entire frequency range when potential to cope and sense of power is high.

Other researchers have shown that in humans, happy voices have been shown to have high variability in loudness and pitch and are high in the first two formant frequencies. For example, research by Kamiloglu and colleagues found that pitch, loudness, and formant features have clear connections with happiness in human voices. In particular, they found that compared with neutral voices, the voices of people expressing happiness were higher in pitch, variability, range, loudness, and means of the first two formats (indicating higher frequency) [KAMILOGLU2021]. Other research has found loud and high-pitched vocalizations to be associated with high arousal emotions such as fear and joy, with low-arousal emotions such as boredom appearing to be lower in pitch and having slower rates of speech [BACHOROWSKI1995; BANSE1996; ZEIPOLLERMANN2002].

VOICE FEATURES AND MENTAL HEALTH

How Stress Affects Voice

Some research has focused on patterns in voice that co-occur with stress. These studies offer insight into the potential mechanisms that relate to the voice-stress response. Due to the various muscular, respiratory, and neural systems involved, we can see how voice production is considered a psychophysiological process that can be influenced by environmental and/or internal stressors [HANSEN2007]. Stress can be related to mental, social, and physical stressors and stressors coming from internal or external conditions (such as noise, extreme temperatures, danger, illness, discomfort, and isolation [HANCOCK2008]). When a stressor occurs, an individual appraises this stressor and their perceived ability to cope and experiences a bidirectional feedback exchange that involves mental effort and physiological responses [LAZARUS1991]. Stress research therefore often does not focus exclusively on the stressor as a unit of analysis, but rather on the reciprocal exchange between an individual and the stressor [HANCOCK2008].

To explore the neurophysiological mechanisms related to stress and voice, the neurovisceral model [THAYER2009] offers helpful perspectives. When a situation is perceived as a stressor, it is related to a subcortical, implicit level of awareness in which a situation is detected as a threat and activates a state of sympathetic arousal [LEDOUX1996; LANE2008]. In a state of alarm, key areas of the brain play an influential role, including the amygdala and its connections to the thalamus, hypothalamus and pituitary, basal ganglia, and brainstem nuclei [LEDOUX1996]. To activate a top-down neural response to help the organism organize itself to adapt to this event, the amygdala bidirectionally communicates with components of the anterior cingulate cortex (ACC), prefrontal cortex, and insula. This cortico-subcortical network plays a major role in innervating the sinoatrial node of the heart via the vagus nerve [VANPUYVELDE2018]. When there are high levels of top-down control from these networks, they are better able to stimulate the inhibitory action of the parasympathetic nervous system modulated by the vagus nerve [LEDOUX1996; LANE2008]. However, in a state of perceived and/or accurately detected emergency, if there is reduced vagal tone and high arousal, these top-down, prefrontal-directed mechanisms shut down, and more automatic processes dominate the response [LANE2008].

This is important to highlight as we continue our exploration of communication, and the relationship between stress and voice. When top-down mechanisms are easily accessible and engaged, this has a regulating response on the organism, which in turn affects its breathing rate, heart rhythms, and muscle tone. As we will continue to see in upcoming sections, this affects various features of the voice. This voice-stress-heart dynamic means that our ability to accurately detect (in a context-sensitive way) and respond to social interactions and other events has a dramatic effect on some of our key biomechanisms for communication, including voice and facial expression. If a person is not able to employ some of these top-down regulatory mechanisms, the communication signals they send may be coming from less-regulated, automatic, and implicit responses to stress. Automatic and implicit responses introduce challenges to adaptive communication. This is because there is less chance for flexibility in the response and a lack of awareness that could help a person choose a different one.

To help us understand how stress influences voice, we can look at three different processes: breathing, phonation (the utterance of speech sounds), and resonance (the quality of voice that results from vocal fold vibrations) [KREIMAN2011]. When we vocalize, we control breathing with respiratory (the thorax and diaphragm) and laryngeal muscles, which are controlled by special efferent (motor) fibers of the vagus nerve [MACLARNON1999; CAMARA2015]. For phonation to occur, there must be a certain amount of pressure of airflow below the glottis or space between the vocal folds, which means there is a coordination of breathing and glottal opening and closing to create a vibration that becomes a voice frequency [ZHANG2015]. In line with this, research on stress and voice reveals that fluctuations in subglottal pressure [YAO2016] and perturbations in the mucous of the vocal folds can lead to stress-related patterns within jitter and shimmer measurements [HIGGINS1989; KREIMAN2011].

Due to its various branches, the vagus nerve also plays a role in the interconnection of these systems involved in breathing, speech, and stress responses [YOSHIDA1992; CAMARA2015; HAMMER2015]. For example, the superior laryngeal nerve acts on the cricothyroid muscle to stretch vocal folds and regulate pitch [KREIMAN2011]. Fibers from the superior laryngeal nerve also split from the vagus nerve and travel through the carotid artery to control intrinsic laryngeal muscles [CAMARA2015]. Finally, all of these processes need to be controlled by changing the shape and positioning of the lips, tongue, larynx, and other parts of the mouth, throat, and jaw in order to shape the vibrations into formant frequencies [CLARK1990; STORY 1998; KREIMAN2011]. Given the complex interplay of stress and all the systems involved in respiration and neuromuscular control, stress can impact any of these aspects of voice production.

Depression and Voice

Due to the complexity of the systems involved, speech can serve as a valuable tool for examining mental health and wellbeing. Even slight physiological and cognitive changes can produce observable acoustic changes [SCHERER1986]. For example, vocal expressions of people with depression have recognizable acoustic patterns of low intensity, less pitch variation, flat speech (monotonicity), and reduced articulation rate [FRANCE2000; MOORE2003; ZLOCHOWER1996]. Voice features have also been used to diagnose depression [ALGHOWINEM2013, MOORE2008; SCHERER2013].

Studies on vocal expression in individuals with depression have revealed a variety of recognizable characteristics, such as low intensity, increased monotonicity (less variation in pitch and flat speech), low articulation rate, and varied pause duration [FRANCE2000; MOORE2003; ZLOCHOWER1996]. Depressed individuals also perform worse when it comes to recognizing discrete emotions from vocal prosody and demonstrate a general bias toward negative emotions and reduced perception of positive prosody [PERON2011; UEKERMANN2008; SCHLIPF2013]. Prosodic features of voice associated with depression have been well documented. Various research studies have found patterns in prosodic abnormalities among depressed subjects, including reduced speaking intensity, reduced pitch range, slower speech rate, reduced intonation, and articulation errors [HOLLIEN1980; CUMMINS2015; NILSONNE1985, 1988]. Fundamental frequency (f0) has also been shown to be affected by a person's mood [ELLGRING1996], level of agitation, and anxiety [ALPERT2001] associated with depression. Speech rate— another prosodic feature—appears in the literature as a promising marker for recognizing depression. Many studies have reported that the rate of speaking in depressed individuals is slower than in controls [DARBY1977; GODFREY1984; GREDEN1980; GREDEN1981; HARDY1984; HOLLIEN1980; SZABADI1976; TEASDALE1980].

Some patterns within voice features such as jitter, shimmer, and harmonic-to-noise ratio have been shown to correlate strongly with depression, psycho-motor retardation (PMR), and suicidality [OZDAS2004A; QUATIERI2012] due to their connection to vocal fold vibration [SUNDBERG2011]. Other research has shown that depression is tied to phonation and articulation errors [CHRISTOPHER2005] and difficulty choosing words [ALPERT20011; MUNDT2012].

Suicidality and Voice

The first observations of voice and speech features associated with suicidality were noted by psychiatrist Dr. S. Silverman as he listened to recorded sessions with suicidal patients and recorded suicide notes [CUMMINS2015; SILVERMAN2010]. These patients were suffering from depression and subsequently attempted suicide. From these investigations, Silverman noted that as an individual becomes presuicidal, changes occur in their speech, including four particular features: hollow tone, decreases in intensity, vocal patterns such as monotony or mechanical phrasing, and unexpected emphasis on certain words or utterances that are not part of normal speech syntax [CUMMINS2015; SILVERMAN2010]. Researchers have also been able to accurately discriminate between male control voices and suicidal voices with an accuracy of 80% using a prediction of flattened speech within spectral density measurements [FRANCE2000]. It is important to note, however, that due to confounding or overlapping symptoms within depression and suicidality, such as anxiety, agitations, fatigue, insomnia, working memory impairments, and low mood, speech-based measurements may indicate voice features for either or both [CUMMINS2015]. This should therefore be considered when using speech analysis to assess these conditions.

Post-traumatic Stress and Voice

Speech analysis has also been explored in the realm of identifying post-traumatic stress disorder (PTSD). Some research has suggested that voice profiles associated with PTSD include increased tension [SCHERER2013] and decreased vowel space [SCHERER2016]. In a study by Charles Marmar and colleagues using artificial intelligence algorithms, several voice features were found to be associated with warzone-exposed veterans diagnosed with PTSD compared to controls, including slower, more monotonous speech, less change in tonality, and less activation (which represents variability in certain speech frequencies) [MARMAR2019].

Anger and Voice

Another type of research explored how expressive vocal behavior influences the experience of anger and cardiovascular reactivity. Two studies found that when participants spoke about anger-arousing and neutral events using different voice styles, differences were found in heart rate reactivity, blood pressure, and reported experiences. The fast and loud speech style was associated with significantly greater blood pressure, significantly higher heart rate reactivity, and reports of feeling significantly angrier compared to normal speaking styles [SIEGMAN1990]. The same participants also showed significantly lower blood pressure reactivity and reported feeling significantly less angry in the slow and soft conditions compared with the normal voice condition [SIEGMAN1990].

Sleep Deprivation and Voice

Sleep deprivation may also be detected in voice. Studies on sleep deprivation have shown links between Sleep, Activity, Fatigue, and Task Effectiveness (SAFTE) and voice acoustics [GREELEY2006; HURSH2004].

INFORMATION CONTAINED IN THE VOICE

The amount of information contained in vocalizations is vast. Some of the aspects of information about a person that has been shown to emerge from voice include:

- Size: receivers can extract body size information from the voice: higher pitch and formant frequencies are related to smaller size in most mammals [PISANSKI2014; TAYLOR2010].

- Gender: human listeners are typically able to infer whether a voice is from a man or woman [ANDREWS1997; BACHOROWSKI1999]. Due to having larger vocal folds, men produce a mean pitch and formants that are on average lower than those produced by women [RENDALL2005].

- Identity: human listeners can accurately identify a specific person and discriminate between individuals from voice [KREIMAN2011]. Voice can also convey other aspects of identity such as regional accents and pronunciation [LAVAN2019].

- Emotion: to understand how emotions are conveyed through voice, it is helpful to explore some of the muscular and physiological changes that occur within the somatic and autonomic nervous systems (the sympathetic and parasympathetic nervous system). We will look at this beginning with the Brunswikian functional lens model.

The Brunswikian Functional Lens Model

The Brunswikian functional lens model is a framework for understanding how internal processes are expressed through vocal signals [BRUNSWIK1952; SCHERER2011]. In this model, a person expresses internal processes in the form of physical signals using their voice. The process includes the following mechanisms:

- The voice producer encodes different types of information (such as their emotional state) via a series of *distal cues*. Distal means "away from the body." These are the patterns of acoustic signals that can be objectively measured.

- When the receiver senses the distal cues using their auditory perceptual mechanisms, these signals become *proximal cues*. Proximal means close to the body. These are the signals that are now captured by the receiver.

- The receiver then makes judgments about the signals they receive via a process called *decoding* or *cue utilization*.

In successful communication, the receiver accurately perceives and infers the information from the cues sent by the producer [KAMILOGLU2021; BRUNSWIK1952; SCHERER2011]. Some studies using principles of this model, including encoding of distal cues, and decoding of proximal cues show some patterns and possible profiles of vocal parameters of different emotions. The following are some of the acoustic profiles that emerged from a study conducted by Banse and Scherer, which replicated findings from many other studies [BANSE1996].

Fundamental frequency (F0): Mean F0 has been shown as being the highest during "intense emotions" of despair, "hot anger,"* panic fear, and elation and lowest for contempt and boredom. It shows up as being in the middle range for happiness, anxiety, shame, ride, sadness, disgust, interest, and "cold anger"* [BANSE1996].

Mean Energy: Mean energy shows relatively high correlations with fundamental frequency and thus similar patterns in emotions. The highest mean energy is shown to be associated with the four "intense" emotions: despair, hot anger, panic fear, and elation. The lowest means in energy have been paired with shame and sadness—which is slightly different than the pattern for fundamental frequency (where they were in the middle range). This may have some connection to a dampening of arousal that we already explored in Chapter 2 related to social referencing and the use of "misattunement" to inhibit exploratory behavior. Another interesting finding emerged from the patterns of mean energy related to vocalizations of disgust and contempt, which showed an acoustic pattern of very low F0 and relatively low energy [BANSE1996]. In animal communication, low F0 is associated with dominance and superiority displays [MORTON1977].

Energy distribution in the spectrum: A finding related to this parameter is worth noting: when it came to sadness, a remarkably high proportion of energy was in the low frequencies as compared with the mean of all other emotions [BANSE1996]. Drawing from the Component Process model, Banse and Scherer assert that the appraisal of having little control over a situation (low coping potential) result in a lax voice with more low-frequency energy and has a stronger influence over physiologic-acoustic changes than the appraisal of a stimulus being pleasant or unpleasant [BANSE1996].

Studies based on the Brunswikian model have also revealed several relational dimensions that emerge from how distal cues (including vocal prosody, emotional expressions, and emotional language) are sent out and received by others [BURGOON2022]:

- **Dominance–Non-Dominance**: A feature of relationships that has a significant influence on behaviors and communication signals is dominance. Dominance reflects the level of power and status of a person who is subservient and whether the dynamic is egalitarian [BURGOON2022]. Micro-level nonverbal and verbal behaviors of dominance include talking more often and for longer duration; lower variability in the harmonic sound of voice can also be perceived as dominance [BURGOON2022; ZHOU2004].

- **Affection-Hostility**: Affection-Hostility can also be phrased as liking-disliking. Various like-dislike behaviors overlap with other expressions such as immediacy [BURGOON2022]. Immediacy is an interplay of vocal, linguistic, kinesic (body movement), and proxemic (spatial separation) features that signal closeness or distance [BURGOON1985, 2022A]. Behaviors associated with liking and affiliation also include a variety of pitch, relaxed laughter, inclusive first-person plurals ("we" and "us"), and positive affect language [BURGOON2022].

- **Involvement-Detachment:** Involvement can have positive or negative connotations and influences the intensity of expressions of dominance and affiliation [DILLARD]. Higher perceived involvement is associated with more words, sentences, and longer turns-at-talk duration, indicating increased participation in group discussion [BURGOON2022]. Higher involvement is also associated with more vocal warmth and relaxation [COKER1987; BURGOON2022].

- **Composure-Nervousness**: Composure is a relational message that conveys that one is comfortable and at ease in the other's presence. Signals of composure include facial and postural relaxation and an acoustically more expressive and pleasant voice, as well as higher average loudness and less hoarseness in the voice (what is called "average shimmer") [BURGOON2022]. The opposite of composure is nervousness. Nervousness can manifest as rigid facial expressions, gaze avoidance, fidgeting, softer vocal amplitude, higher pitch, shorter and fewer turns-at-talk [BURGOON2021, 2022]. Nervousness is shown particularly in the upper and lower action units of the face, such as the brow, eye, lip, and chin regions [BURGOON2022].

- **Trust-Distrust**: Trust increases cooperation [BALLIET2013] and reduces the risks and costs of social transactions [DYER2003]. Using a variety of definitions and studies, some foundational features of trust include benevolence, integrity, competence, and predictability are seen as underlying [MCKNIGHT2000]. Other verbal and nonverbal cues are associated with trust, such as smile [CENTORRINO2015], eye contact or gaze aversion [BAYLISS2006], facial expressivity [KRUMHUBER2007], voice pitch [MCALEER2014], prosody dynamics [CHEN2020]. Less hoarse voice and less breathiness can stimulate trust [BURGOON2022]. Conversely, high levels of "adaptor behavior" such as brow-lowering, lip-sucking have been found to diminish trust [BURGOON2022].

Voice production and reception play an important role in communication. Understanding the muscular configurations offers an opportunity to have more intentional control over the quality, amplitude, pitch, and intensity of our voice. It also opens opportunities for objective, measurable, physiological measurements for detecting features and profiles associated with various mental health conditions. As we will see in the section on middle ear muscles, the frequencies we detect in our environment and from other people have effects on our internal state. These interactions of muscular movements create frequencies (whether audible from voice, or visible frequencies such as in facial expressions, or using hands to create graphical symbols such as words), and our reception of these frequencies forms the basis of communication feedback systems. While all mammals use vocalization for communication, humans have an increased degree of complexity for the variety of voice and face expressions due to muscular and other physical attributes of the tongue, vocal folds and other muscles in the face and head. Moreover, what we see from the above research is that a person's internal state and underlying mental health affect the dimensions and amount of information available to be transmitted to another person. Variability of pitch, frequency, loudness, tone, etc., reveal ongoing, emergent fluctuations in each person's internal state and intention. The more information we are able to transmit and receive using our various methods of nonverbal and verbal communication, the more accurately we can assess the best next action to take within each interaction. As we will see in the next section, the frequencies that we detect within our environment and social interactions add an important dimension to our communicative feedback system.

PERCEIVING VOICE

Another element of communication and the social engagement system is related to our mechanisms for perceiving sounds in our environment—with a specialized system for detecting human voices amidst all the other sounds that are around us. Humans use their voice for both verbal and nonverbal strategies for sending out signals to convey information and influence others' behaviors. In the past, hearing was theorized to be an entirely passive process [GILMOR1989]. In the late 1940s, this theory was updated by French hearing loss and voice expert, Alfred Tomatis, who proposed alternative theories about the active role of the middle ear in the processes needed for listening. He proposed that, just as the eye can shift from passively seeing to actively looking, the ear can also shift from passively hearing to actively listening and that this process of listening is both motivational and neurophysiological [GILMOR1989]. His theory came about through several breakthroughs that occurred during his work on assessing industrial hearing loss in ammunition factory workers, as well as his private practice treatment of opera singers who had voice problems [GILMOR1989]. This work led him to discover significant hearing loss in factory workers, especially the higher frequency ranges, as well as complaints of fatigue, irritability, and poor quality of voice and speech [GILMOR1989]. He also found these similar symptoms of irritability and fatigue in opera singers with vocal problems who were not responding well to the usual treatments, which led him to discover a high correspondence between the voice and the ear: the voice can only reproduce sounds that the ear can hear. The opera singers' voice difficulties were hearing-related. He then began to experiment with amplifiers and filters to enhance or modify certain frequencies [GILMOR1989]. As the singers heard themselves with modified frequencies, their voices improved. Tomatis also found that constant training of the ear led to lasting improvements for the singers, which led to what is called the "Law of Retention" [GILMOR1989]. Further discoveries were made on how the middle ear and facial muscles can influence the quality of the listening response of the ear, which can then modify the quality of the voice [TOMATIS1974]. These discoveries increased our understanding of how the auditory system filters frequencies through middle ear mechanisms.

Sound Frequencies and Nervous System Responses

Our environments are filled with vast amounts of frequencies that can be picked up by various mechanisms within our auditory system. Sounds coming from potential threats activate various defense mechanisms including the commonly known mobilization tactic of fight-or-flight, as well as other strategies including immobilization [PORGES2021]. Sights, sounds, smells, and other sensory inputs detected as potential threats can represent environmental dangers such as weather (lightning, wind, etc.), as well as other species and machines. Threats also come in the form of other humans, whether they pose a physical threat or a threat in terms of impeding our ability to achieve our goal of homeostasis. Because human communication is a behavioral transmitter and can influence the internal state of another person, threats can also come in the form of verbal strategies such as aggression, bullying, manipulation, and coercion. In contrast to the activation of defense strategies, sounds from the environment and other humans can also initiate nervous system regulation. Our auditory system connects outside sounds to our internal state. The ear, and in particular, the middle ear, plays an important role in human communication and translating external frequencies into electrical input for the brain to process and interpret.

Physiology of the Middle Ear

Sound waves enter the outer ear and travel through the middle ear, and into the inner ear—where sound input can be communicated to the brain. The middle ear has several components that transduce the sound energy from outside into different forms of energy that serve as information for the brain to process.

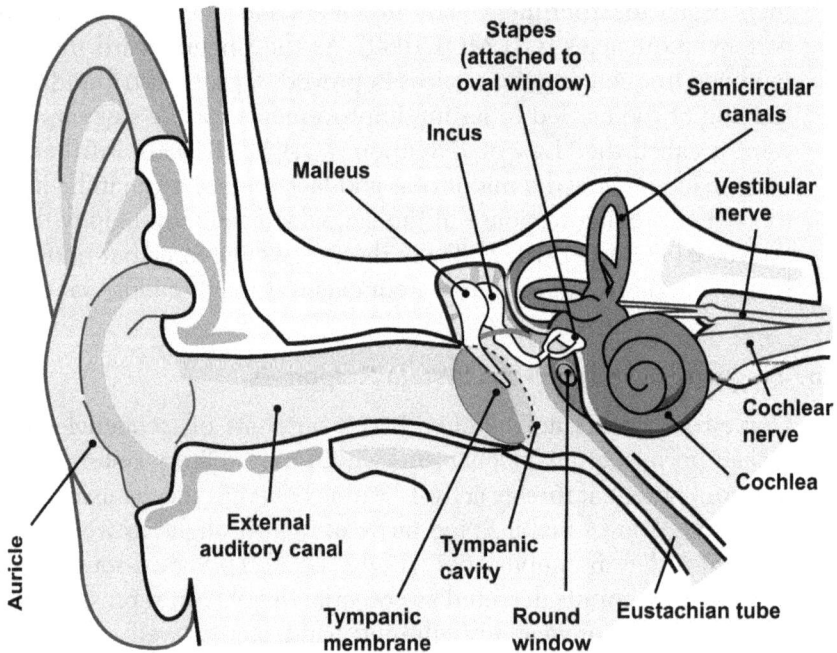

FIGURE 6.2

To understand this journey, we will look at the various components of the middle ear. The middle ear has different parts that each serve their own function:

- Tympanic membrane (the eardrum)
- Tympanic cavity
- Middle ear muscles
- Ossicles
- Auditory (eustachian) tube

The tympanic membrane is also known as the eardrum and separates the middle ear from the external ear. It is semitransparent and has a tense portion called the *pars tensa* (where it gets stretched tight, much like the skin on a drum) and a loose section that is more flaccid, called the *pars flaccida* [SPENCER2016]. In the following section, we will see why this tightening and stretching is important for understanding our perception of threat and how it affects our internal state.

The tympanic cavity is a rectangular space with four walls, a ceiling, and a floor, with the lateral consisting of the tympanic membrane. The floor separates the middle ear from the jugular vein. Within the anterior wall of this structure are two openings—one for the auditory tube and the other for the tensor tympani (one of the middle ear muscles). The two muscles of the middle ear are the tympani and stapedius. The tensor tympani helps protect the ear from loud sounds by tensing the tympanic membrane to reduce the amplitude of oscillations [SPENCER2016]. The stapedius is a tiny muscle that also helps reduce the loudness of sound by contracting the stapes, and thereby minimizing vibrations traveling to the cochlea via the oval window. The stapedius is connected to a small branch of the facial nerve [GAILLARD2008].

The ossicles are tiny bones in the middle ear making up the ossicular chain, which consists of the malleus (hammer), the incus (anvil), and the stapes (stirrup). Sound waves are funneled into the outer ear and are carried through the middle ear, where they hit the tympanic membrane. As they hit the eardrum, they cause a vibration that sets the three ossicles in motion and further amplifies the sound [HOPKINS2023]. The stapes bone is attached to the oval window. The vibrations from the oval window travel into the inner ear, where fluid inside the cochlea moves and sets many nerve endings into motion. These nerve endings then transduce the vibrations into electrical impulses that travel up to the brain via the auditory nerve and are interpreted by the brain [HOPKINS2023].

The middle ear plays a key role in adjusting our perception of sound. It does this through the actions of the muscles adjusting the positions of the bones to adjust pressures and tensions within various structures. These adjustments not only protect the ear from sudden loud sounds, but they also promote an active process of listening through a constant telescope-like adjustment to accommodate a spectrum of frequencies [GILMOR1989].

In this way, the middle ear muscles extract human speech by dampening low-frequency sounds from the environment and allowing higher frequencies to transmit to the inner ear [PORGES2021]. This mechanism occurs through how the middle ear muscles influence the tightness or looseness of the eardrum. They do this by regulating the tiny bones within the ossicular chain. The rigidity of the ossicular chain influences the stiffness of the eardrum. The middle ear muscles modulate the position of the ossicles, which stiffens or loosens the membrane of the eardrum. When the eardrum tightens, lower frequencies are reflected and therefore attenuated before being transmitted to the inner ear. As it dampens lower frequencies, the tightening of the eardrum also allows higher frequencies to be absorbed and transmitted to the inner ear (cochlea) and then further transmitted to the brain (cortex) via the auditory nerve (cranial nerve VII) [PORGES2021]. An important function of the middle ear is therefore to dampen background sounds from low frequencies. These can be from things like ventilation and heating systems, traffic, appliances, and airplanes. The tightening of the ossicular chain is also part of how humans extract the human voice from all the other sounds that exist in our environment. If we are at a coffee shop having a conversation, for example, the middle ear muscles are working to muffle or dampen all the other sounds around us in order for us to pick up on the frequencies of the person speaking.

The following neurophysiological principles play a role in how the neural mechanisms regulate the middle ear muscles as they interact with specific bands and frequencies of acoustic energies [PORGES2021]:

- The middle ear dampens low-frequency sounds and helps extract frequencies of human voice from background noise [PORGES2021].

- Acoustic energy is transmitted across middle ear structures to middle ear muscles regardless of tone at a resonance frequency between 800 to 1200 Hz in children [HANKS1993].

- Middle ear muscles are made up of fast-twitch muscle fibers and are susceptible to fatigue [SCHIAFFINO2011].

■ Middle ear muscles are linked with a brainstem area that is also tied to the regulation of striated muscles of the face and head [PORGES2021].

Understanding the active role of the middle ear and its muscles also offers insight into why children with a history of ear infections are at higher risk of language and learning disorders [KATZ1978]. When the ear is infected, the fluid build-up can lead to immobilization of the muscles in the middle ear. Like any muscle, these tiny muscles can also become weak with disuse. Children with genetic or neurological conditions associated with poor muscle tone or control (Down syndrome and cerebral palsy) also often demonstrate challenges in listening and concentrating [GILMOR1989]. Moreover, lack of middle ear muscle tone may also offer insight into auditory hypersensitivity, where the middle ear is less able to tighten and adjust in order to protect the ear from unwanted sound [GILMOR1989].

Perception of Voices and Mental Health

Some research has explored brain activation in response to varying sound intensities and emotional prosody. A study using event-related functional magnetic resonance imaging revealed that people with Social Anxiety Disorder (SAD) had greater insula activation to loud versus normal voices and more activation in the orbitofrontal cortex in response to angry versus neutral prosody compared with healthy controls [SIMON2017]. Moreover, those with SAD also showed greater amygdala activation to loud, angry voices than the control group. The researchers suggest that these results show that voice sound intensity has a modulating effect on amygdala hyperresponsivity to angry prosody in people with SAD. This further suggests that in SADs, the amygdala may engage in abnormal processing of threat signals not only for facial expressions but also for voice [SIMON2017].

The perception of prosody appears to be affected by certain conditions such as depression and schizophrenia. In studies exploring the perception of emotional prosody, individuals with depression show a negativity bias in their perception of emotions [KAN2004], reduced perception of positive prosody [SCHLIPF2013] and perform worse in recognition of discrete emotions compared with healthy controls [PERON2011; UEKERMANN2008]. Individuals with schizophrenia demonstrate difficulty in recognizing emotions based on others' voices [HOEKERT2007; LEITMAN2018].

These studies suggest a relationship between mental health challenges and the ability to accurately perceive nuanced emotional information from vocal prosody. These findings could have important implications for many professions, including police and first responders, as well as clinicians and teaching professionals. This also applies to family dynamics. The human perception of voice signals and facial expressions can be skewed by existing mental health challenges, and other conditions that may activate brain networks and responses that lower the person's context sensitivity. This means they may perceive signals within an interaction as more threatening than is appropriate or adaptive for the context. This can lead to their own defensive strategies that feed into the subsequent appraisals and behaviors of the other person in that dyad or group. Awareness of these mechanisms offers an opportunity for people to adjust their own responses. For example, if we are dealing with a person who appears to be perceiving our behavior as threatening, and we understand how our voice and facial gestures may be skewed heavily toward threat, we could experiment with adjusting the emotional prosody and sound intensity of our voice to see if this creates a change in their response.

Vocal Expressions of Positive Emotions

Several studies suggest that emotion-specific patterns of acoustic features exist for differentiated and discrete negative emotions such as anger, fear, and sadness [BANSE1996]. Research is also revealing differentiations between positive emotional states. For example, happy voices have been found to be generally loud with a high amount of variability in loudness and pitch and are high in the first two formant frequencies [KAMILOGLU2021]. Further pattern mapping of positive emotions comparing pitch, loudness, and speech rate also suggests emotion families. For example, amusement, interest, and relief are considered epistemological emotions[2] and are associated with a higher pitch, while contentment and pleasure are clustered as savoring emotions and are more moderate in pitch [KAMILOGLU2021].

SUMMARY

In this chapter, we explored some of the mechanisms involved in voice production, as well as mechanisms related to hearing and listening. We saw that various features of voice may be influenced by mental health conditions. We also examined how various nervous system components, respiration,

---

[2] Epistemic or epistemological is a term related to knowledge or knowing. Epistemic emotions may include surprise, curious, confusion, amusement, interest, and relief [VOGL2020].

and vocal parameters are involved in conveying our internal state. Voice frequencies and facial gestures convey important information and can influence the internal state and behaviors of others. While these nonverbal elements of communication offer a rich spectrum of information and avenues for an understanding of how much we are affected by others' faces and voices, our next dimension of exploration is within the verbal realm. In addition to facial and vocal configurations, humans also have access to other methods of adding information to our communicative interactions: words, gestures, and symbols, the topic of Chapter 7. In Chapter 8, we will take a look at how language plays a role in developing executive functioning, maturity, and social understanding.

REFERENCES

[ABHANG2016] Abhang, P. A., Gawali, B. W., and Mehrotra, S. C. (2016). *Introduction to EEG- and speech-based emotion recognition.* Academic Press: San Francisco.

[ADOLPHS2018] Adolphs, R., and Anderson, D. J. (2018). *The neuroscience of emotion: A new synthesis.* Princeton, NJ: Princeton University Press.

[ALPERT2001] Alpert, M., Pouget, E. R., and Silva, R. R. (2001). Reflections of depression in acoustic measures of the patient's speech. *Journal of Affective Disorders 66,* 59–69.

[ANDREWS1997] Andrews, M. L., and Schmidt, C. P. (1997). Gender presentation: Perceptual and acoustical analyses of voice. *Journal of Voice, 11,* 307–313.

[ANIKIN2020] Anikin, A. (2020). A moan of pleasure should be breathy: The effect of voice quality on the meaning of human nonverbal vocalizations. *Phonetica, 77*(5), 327–349.

[BACHOROWSKI1995] Bachorowski, J. A., and Owren, M. J. (1995). Vocal expression of emotion: Acoustic properties of speech are associated with emotional intensity and context. *Psychological Science, 6,* 219–224.

[BACHOROWSKI1999] Bachorowski, J. A., and Owren, M. J. (1999). Acoustic correlates of talker sex and individual talker identity are present in a short vowel segment produced in running speech. *The Journal of the Acoustical Society of America, 106,* 1054–1063.

[BADDELEY2003]. Baddeley, A. (2003). Working memory and language: an overview. *The Journal of Communication Disorders, (36)*, 189–208.

[BALLIET2013] Balliet, D., and Van Lange, P. A. (2013). Trust, conflict, and cooperation: A meta-analysis. *Psychological Bulletin, 139*, 1090–1112.

[BANSE1996] Banse, R., and Scherer, K. (1996). Acoustic profiles in vocal emotion expression. *Journal of Personality and Social Psychology*, 70(3), 614–636.

[BAYLISS2006] Bayliss, A. P., and Tipper, S. P. (2006). Predictive gaze cues and personality judgments: Should eye trust you? *Psychological Science, 17*, 514–520.

[BENWARD1997/2003] Benward, Bruce and Saker, Marilyn (1997/2003). *Music: In Theory and Practice*, Vol. I, 7th ed.; p. xiii. McGraw-Hill. ISBN 978-0-07-294262-0.

[BERLIN2004] Berlin, P., Fecteau, S., and Bedard, C. (2004). Thinking the voice: Neural correlates of voice perception. *Trends in Cognitive Sciences, (8)*, 129–125.

[BERNTSON1991] Berntson, G. G., Cacioppo, J. T., and Quigley, K. S. (1991). Autonomic determinism: the modes of autonomic control, the doctrine of autonomic space, and the laws of autonomic constraint. *Psychological Review (98)*, 459–487.

[BOUCSEIN1992] Boucsein, W. (1992). *Electrodermal Activity*. New York, NY: Plenum Press.

[BREIMAN2001] Breiman, L. (2001). Random forests. *Machine Learning, 45(1)*, 5–32.

[BRUNSWIK1952] Brunswick, E. (1952). *The conceptual framework of psychology*. Chicago: Chicago University Press.

[BRUDZYNSKI2010] Brudzynski, S. M. (Ed.) (2010) *Handbook of Mammalian Vocalization: An Integrative Neuroscience Approach*. San Diego: Academic Press.

[BURGOON1985] Burgoon, J. K., Manusov, V., Mineo, P., and Hale, J. L. (1985). Effects of eye gaze on hiring, credibility, attraction and relational message interpretation. *The Journal of Nonverbal Behavior, 9*, 133–146.

[BURGOON2022] Burgoon, J. K., Wang, R. X., Chen, X., Ge, T. S., and Dorn, B. (2022). How the Brunswikian lens model illustrates the relationship between physiological and behavioral signals and psychological emotional and cognitive states. *Frontiers in Psychology, 12,* 781487. DOI: 10.3389/fpsyg.2021.781487.

[BURGOON2022A]. Burgoon, J. K., Manusov, V., and Guerrero, L. K. (2022). *Nonverbal Communication*, 2nd ed. London: Routledge.

[CAMARA2015] Câmara, R., and Griessenauer, C. J. (2015). Anatomy of the vagus nerve. *Nerves Nerve Injection, 1,* 385–397. doi: 10.1016/B978-0-12-410390-0.00028-7

[CENTORRINO2015] Centorrino, S., Djemai, E., Hopfensitz, A., Milinski, M., and Seabright, P. (2015). Honest signaling in trust interactions: smiles rated as genuine induce trust and signal higher earning opportunities. *Evolution and Human Behavior, 36,* 8–16.

[CHEN2020] Chen, X. L., Ita Levitan, S., Levine, M., Mandic, M., and Hirschberg, J. (2020). Acoustic-prosodic and lexical cues to deception and trust: deciphering how people detect lies. *Transactions of the Association for Computational Linguistics, 8,* 199–214.

[CHRISTOPHER2005] Christopher, G., and MacDonald, J. (2005). The impact of clinical depression on working memory. *Cognitive Neuropsychology, 10,* 379–399.

[CLARK1990] Clark, J., and Yallop, C. (1990). *An Introduction to Phonetics & Phonology*. Oxford: Basil Blackwell.

[COKER1987] Coker, D. A., and Burgoon, J. (1987). The nature of conversational involvement and nonverbal encoding patterns. *Human Communication Research, (13),* 463–494.

[CONSTANINI2006] Costantini, F., and D'Amato, F. R. (2006). Ultrasonic vocalizations in mice and rats: social contexts and functions. *Acta Zoologica Sinica 52,* 619–633.

[COSMIDES1983] Cosmides, L. (1983). Invariances in the acoustic expression of emotion during speech. *Journal of Experimental Psychology: Human Perception and Performance,* 9(6), 864–881.

[CUMMINS2013a] Cummins, N., Epps, J., and Ambikairajah, E. (2013a). Spectro-temporal analysis of speech affected by depression and psychomotor retardation. *Proceedings of 2013 IEEE International Conference on Acoustics, Speech and Signal Processing*, Vancouver, Canada, pp. 7542–7546, doi: 10.1109/ICASSP.2013.6639129.

N. Cummins, J. Epps and E. Ambikairajah, "Spectro-temporal analysis of speech affected by depression and psychomotor retardation," 2013 IEEE International Conference on Acoustics, Speech and Signal Processing, Vancouver, BC, Canada, 2013, pp. 7542-7546, doi: 10.1109/ICASSP.2013.6639129.

[CUMMINS2015] Cummins, N., Scherer, S., Krajewski, J., Schnieder, S., Epps, J., and Quatieri, T. F. (2015). A review of depression and suicide risk assessment using speech analysis. *Speech Communication, 71*, 10–49. *https://doi.org/10.1016/j.specom.2015.03.004*

[DARBY1984] Darby, J. K., Simmons, N., and Berger, P. A. (1984). Speech and voice parameters of depression: A pilot study. *The Journal of Communication Disorders, 17*, 75–85.

[DEBOER2019] De Boer, B. (2019). Evolution of speech: Anatomy and control. *Journal of Speech, Language and Hearing Research, 62(85)*, 2932–2945.

[DEMARTSEV2022] Demartsev, V., Manser, M. B., and Tattersall, G. J. (2022). Vocalization-associated respiration patterns: thermography-based monitoring and detection of preparation for calling. *The Journal of Experimental Biology, 225(5)*, jeb243474. *https://doi.org/10.1242/jeb.243474*

[DEMENKO2012] Demenko, G., and Jastrzêbska, M. (2012). Analysis of natural speech under stress. *Acta Physica Polonica series A General Physics, 121*, A92.

[DILLARD1999] Dillard, J. P., Solomon, D. H., and Palmer, M. T. (1999). Structuring the concept of relational communication. *Communication Monographs, 66*, 49–65.

[DYER2003] Dyer, J. H., and Chu, W. (2003). The role of trustworthiness in reducing transaction costs and improving performance: empirical evidence from the United States, Japan, and Korea. *Organization Science, 14*, 57–68.

[ELLGRING1996] Ellgring, H., and Scherer, K. (1996). Vocal indicators of mood change in depression. *The Journal of Nonverbal Behavior, 20*, 83–110.

[ELLIS1989]. Ellis, A. W. (1989). Neuro-cognitive processing of faces and voices. In H.D. Young and A. W. Ellis (Eds.), *Handbook of Research on Face Processing* (pp. 207–215). Amsterdam, The Netherlands: Elsevier Science Publications B.V.

[ESLING2019] Esling, J., Moisik, S., Benner, A., and Crevier-Buchman, L. (2019). *Voice Quality: The Laryngeal Articulator Model.* New York: Cambridge University Press.

[FANT1960]. Fant, G. (1960). *Acoustic Theory of Speech Production.* The Hague, The Netherlands: Mouton and Co.

[FERNANDES2018] Fernandes, J., Teixeira, F. Guedes, V., Junior, A., and Teixeira, J. P. (2018). Harmonic to noise ratio measurement – Selection of window and length. *Proceida Computer Science (138)*, 280–285.

[FITCH2000] Fitch, W. T. (2000). The evolution of speech: A comprehensive review. *Trends in Cognitive Sciences (4)*, 259–267.

[FITCH2018] Fitch, W. T. (2018). The biology and evolution of speech: A comparative analysis. *Annual Review of Linguistics (4)*, 255–279.

[FRANCE2000] France, D. J., Shiavi, R. G., Silverman, S., Silverman, M., and Wilkes, M. (2000). Acoustical properties of speech as indicators of depression and suicidal risk. *IEEE Transactions on Biomedical Engineering (47)*, 829–837.

[FRICK1985] Frick, R. W. (1985). Communicating emotion: the role of prosodic features, *Psychological Bulletin (97)*, 412–429.

[GAILLARD2008] Gaillard, F., Bell, D., Hacking, C., et al. Stapedius muscle. Reference article, Radiopaedia.org (Accessed on 01 Mar 2023) *https://doi.org/10.53347/rID-2083*

[GILMOR1989] Gilmor, T. M. The Tomatis method and the genesis of listening author. *PhD Pre- and Peri-natal Psychology Journal, 4(1)*, 9–26.

[GOBL2010] Gobl, C., and Chasaide, A. N. (2010). Voice source variation and its communicative functions. In W. J. Hardcastl , J. Laver, & F. E. Gibbon (Eds.), *The Handbook of Phonetic Sciences* (pp. 378–423). Malden, MA: Wiley-Blackwell.

[GODFREY1984] Godfrey, H. P., and Knight, R. G. (1984). The validity of actometer and speech activity measures in the assessment of depressed patients. *The British Journal of Psychiatry, 145*, 159–163.

[GREDEN1980] Greden, J. F., and Carroll, B. J. (1980). Decrease in speech pause times with treatment of endogenous depression. *Biological Psychiatry, 15*, 575–587.

[GREDEN1981] Greden, J. F., Albala, A. A., and Smokler, I. A. (1981). Speech pause time: a marker of psychomotor retardation among endogenous depressives. *Biological Psychiatry, 16*, 851–859.

[GREELEY2006] Greeley, H. P., Friets, E., Wilson, J. P., Raghavan, S., Picone, J., and Berg, J. (2006). Detecting fatigue from voice using speech recognition. In *Proceedings of the IEEE International Symposium on Signal Processing and Information Technology* (Louisville, KY: IEEE), pp. 567–571. doi: 10.1109/ISSPIT.2006.27 0865

[GRICHKOVTSOVA2012] Grichkovtsova, I., Morel, M., and Lacheret, A. (2012). The role of voice quality and prosodic contour in affective speech perception. *Speech Communication, 54*, 414–429.

[HAMMER2015]. Hammer, N., Glätzner, J., Feja, C., Kühne, C., Meixensberger, J., Planitzer, U., et al. (2015). Human vagus nerve branching in the cervical region. *PLoS One* 10:e0118006. doi: 10.1371/journal.pone.0118006

[HANCOCK2008]. Hancock, P. A., and Szalma, J. L. (2008). *Performance Under Stress*. Farnham: Ashgate Publishing, Ltd.

[HANSEN2007]. Hansen, J. H., and Patil, S. (2007). Speech under stress: Analysis, modeling and recognition. In *Speaker Classification I. Lecture Notes in Computer Science, (4343)*, ed. C. Müller (Berlin: Springer), 108–137.

[HARDY1984] Hardy, P., Jouvent, R., and Widloecher, D (1984). Speech pause time and the retardation rating scale for depression (ERD): towards a reciprocal validation. *The Journal of Affective Disorders, 6*, 123–127.

[HIGGINS1989] Higgins, M. B., and Saxman, J. H. (1989). Variations in vocal frequency perturbation across the menstrual cycle. *The Journal of Voice, 3*, 233–243.

[HOEKERT2007] Hoekert, M., Kahn, R., Pijnenborg, M., and Aleman, A. (2007). Impaired recognition and expression of emotional prosody in schizophrenia: Review and meta-analysis . *Schizophrenia Research, 96*, 135–145.

[HOLLIEN1980] Hollien, H. (1980). Vocal indicators of psychological stress. *Annals of the New York Academy of Sciences, 347*, 47–72.

[HOPKINS2023] How the ear works, date of access July 2, 2023 *https://www. hopkinsmedicine.org/health/conditions-and-diseases/how-the-ear-works*

[HURSH2004] Hursh, S. R., Redmond, D. P., Johnson, M. L., Thorne, D. R., Belenky, G., Balkin, T. J., et al. (2004). Fatigue models for applied research in warfighting. *Aerospace Medicine and Human Performance, 75*, A44–A53.

[KAMILOGLU2021] Kamiloglu, R. G., and Sauter, D. A. (2021). Voice production and perception. In O. Braddick (Ed.), *Oxford Research Encyclopedia of Psychology [e-766]*. New York: Oxford University Press.

[KAN2004] Kan, Y., Mimura, M., Kamijima, K., and Kawamura, M. (2004). Recognition of emotion from moving facial and prosodic stimuli in depressed patients. *Journal of Neurology, Neurosurgery and Psychiatry, 75*, 1667–1671.

[KATZ1978] Katz, J. (1978). The effects of conductive hearing loss on auditory function. *ASHA, (10)*, 879–886.

[KENT2000]. Kent, R. D. (2000). Research on speech motor control and its disorders: A review and prospective. *Journal of Communication Disorders, 33(5)*, 391–427.

[KISTLER1998] Kistler, A., Mariauzouls, C., and von Berlepsch, K. (1998). Fingertip temperature as an indicator for sympathetic responses. *The International Journal of Psychophysiology, 29*, 35–41.

[KLOFSTAD2015] Klofstad, C. A., Anderson, R. C., and Nowicki, S. (2015). Perceptions of competence, strength, and age influence voters to select leaders with lower-pitched voices . *PLOS One, 10*, e0133779.

[KRAEPELIN1921] Kraepelin, E. (1921). Manic depressive insanity and paranoia. *The Journal of Nervous and Mental Disease, 53(4)*, 350.

[KREIBIG2010] Kreibig, S. D. (2010). Autonomic nervous system activity in emotion: A review. *Biological Psychology, 84(3)*, 394–421. *https://doi. org/10.1016/j.biopsycho.2010.03.010*

[KREIMAN2011]. Kreiman, J., and Sidtis, D. (2011). *Foundations of Voice Studies: An Interdisciplinary Approach to Voice Production and Perception*. Hoboken, NJ: John Wiley & Sons. doi: 10.1002/9781444395068.

[KRUMHUBER2007] Krumhuber, E., Manstead, A. S., Cosker, D., Marshall, D., Rosin, P. L., and Kappas, A. (2007). Facial dynamics as indicators of trustworthiness and cooperative behavior. *Emotion* 7, 730–735.

[KURAOKA2010] Kuraoka, K. and Nakamura, K. (2010). Chapter 5.3: Vocalization as a specific trigger of emotional responses. In Brudzynski, S. M. (Ed.) *Handbook of Mammalian Vocalization: An Integrative Neuroscience Approach*, Academic Press, San Diego: 2010.

[LABORDE2017] Laborde, S., Mosley, E., and Thayer, J. F. (2017). Heart Rate Variability and Cardiac Vagal Tone in Psychophysiological Research - Recommendations for Experiment Planning, Data Analysis, and Data Reporting. *Frontiers in psychology*, 8, 213. *https://doi. org/10.3389/fpsyg.2017.00213*

[LANE2008] Lane, R. D. (2008). Neural substrates of implicit and explicit emotional processes: a unifying framework for psychosomatic medicine. *Psychosomatic Medicine, 70*, 214–231.

[LAVAN2019] Lavan, N., Burton, A. M., Scott, S. K., and McGettigan, C. (2019). Flexible voices: Identity perception from variable vocal signals. *Psychonomic Bulletin & Review, 26*, 90–102.

[LAZARUS1991] Lazarus, R. S. (1991). *Emotion and Adaptation.* Oxford England: Oxford University Press.

[LEDOUX1996] LeDoux, J. E. (1996). *The Emotional Brain: The Mysterious Underpinnings of Emotional Life*. New York, NY: Simon & Schuster.

[LEITMAN2018] Leitman, D. I., and Haigh, S. M. (2018). Impairments in decoding vocal emotion in schizophrenia and bipolar disorder . In S. Frühholz & P. Belin (Eds.), *The Oxford Handbook of Voice Perception* (pp. 800–830). Oxford England: Oxford University Press.

[LESTER1988] Lester, B. M., and Zeskin, P. S. (1982). A biobehavioral perspective on crying in early infancy. In: Fizgerald, H. , Lester, B. , Yogman, M. (Eds.), *Theory and Research in Behavioral Pediatrics* (pp. 133–180). New York, NY: Plenum Press.

[LEVANGIE2005] Levangie, P. K., and Norkin, C. C. (2005). *Joint structure and function: A comprehensive analysis*, 4th Edn, Philadelphia: FA Davis Publishers (*https://www.physio-pedia.com/ Muscles_of_Respiration#cite_note-strong-1*)

[LIEBERMAN1969] Lieberman, P. H., Klatt, D. H., and Wilson, W. H. (1969). Vocal tract limitations on the vowel repertoires of rhesus monkey and other nonhuman primates. *Science, 164* (3884), 1185–1187.

[LIEBERMAN1988] Lieberman, P., and Blumstein, Se.E. (1988). *Speech Physiology, Speech Perception, And Acoustic Phonetics*. Cambridge: Cambridge University Press.

[LITVIN2007] Litvin, Y., Blanchard, D. C., and Blanchard, R. J., (2007). Rat 22 kHz ultrasonic vocalizations as alarm cries. *Behavioural Brain Research, 182*, 166–172.

[LORENZA2017] Colzato, L. S., Sellaro, R., and Beste, C. (2017). Darwin revisited: The vagus nerve is a causal element in controlling recognition of other's emotions. *Cortex, (92)*, 95–102.

[LUMEN2021] NSCC and Lumen/OpenStax (2021). *Fundamentals of Heat, Light & Sound,* licensed under a Creative Commons Attribution 4.0 International License.

[MACLARNON1999] MacLarnon, A., and Hewitt, G. (1999). The evolution of human speech: the role of enhanced breathing control. *The American Journal of Biological Anthropology, 109*, 341–363. doi: 10.1002/(SICI)1096-8644(199907)109:3<341::AID-AJPA5>3.0.CO;2-2

[MARLER1977] Marler, P., and Tenaza, R. (1977). Signaling behavior of apes with special reference to vocalization. In T.A. Sebeok (Ed.) *How Animals Communicate*, Bloomington, IN: Indiana University Press.

[MARMAR2019] Marmar, C. R., Brown, A. D., Qian, M., Laska, E., Siegel, C., Li, M., Abu-Amara, D., Tsiartas, A., Richey, C., Smith, J., Knoth, B., and Vergyri, D. (2019) Speech-based markers for posttraumatic stress disorder in US veterans. *Depress Anxiety, Jul;36(7)*, 607–616.

[MCALEER2014] McAleer, P., Todorov, A., and Belin, P. (2014). How do you say 'hello'? Personality impressions from brief novel voices. *PLoS One 9*, e90779.

[MCKNIGHT2000] McKnight, D. H., and Chervany, N. L. (2000). What is trust? A conceptual analysis and an interdisciplinary model. In *Proceedings of the AMCIS Americas Conference on Information Systems*, Vol. 382, (Long Beach, CA: AMCIS), 827–833.

[MOORE2008] Moore II, E., Clements, M. A., Peifer, J. W., and Weisser, L. (2008). Critical analysis of the impact of glottal features in the classification of clinical depression in speech. *IEEE Transactions on Biomedical Engineering, 55(1),* 96–107.

[MORTON1977] Morton, E. S. (1977). On the occurrence and significance of motivation-structural rules in some bird and mammal sounds. *American Naturalist, 111,* 855–869.

[MUNDT2012] Mundt, J. C., Vogel, A. P., Feltner, D. E., and Lenderking, W. R. (2012). Vocal acoustic biomarkers of depression severity and treatment response. *Biological Psychiatry, 72(7),* 580–587. *https://doi.org/10.1016/j. biopsych.2012.03.015*

[NEWMAN1938] Newman, S., and Mather, V. G. (1938). Analysis of spoken language of patients with affective disorders. *American Journal of Psychiatry, 94(4),* 913–942. *https://doi.org/10.1176/ajp.94.4.913*

[NILSONNE1985] Nilsonne, A., Sundberg, J., (1985). Differences in ability of musicians and nonmusicians to judge emotional state from the fundamental frequency of voice samples. *Music Percept. 2,* 507–516.

[NILSONNE1988] Nilsonne, A., (1988). Speech characteristics as indicators of depressive illness. *Acta Psychiatrica Scandinavica, 77,* 253–263.

[NITSCHKE1982] Nitschke, W. (1982). *Acoustic Behavior in the Rat. Research, Theory, and Applications.* New York, NY: Praeger Publishers.

[NYBY2010] Nyby, J. G. (2010). Chapter 7.6: Adult house mouse (*Mus musculus*) ultrasonic calls: hormonal and pheromonal regulation, in Brudzynski, S. M. (Ed.) *Handbook of Mammalian Vocalization: An Integrative Neuroscience Approach.* San Diego: Academic Press.

[OZDAS2004A] Ozdas, A., Shiavi, R. G., Silverman, S. E., Silverman, M. K., and Wilkes, D. M. (2004a). Investigation of vocal jitter and glottal flow spectrum as possible cues for depression and near-term suicidal risk. *IEEE Transactions on Biomedical Engineering, 51,* 1530–1540.

[PANSKEPP2000] Panksepp, J., and Burgdorf, J. (2000). 50-kHz chirping (laughter?) in response to conditioned and unconditioned tickle induced reward in rats: effects of social housing and genetic variables. *Behavioural Brain Research, 115,* 25–38.

[PERON2011] Peron, J., El Tamer, S, Grandjean, D., Leray, E., Travers, D., Drapier, D., Verin, M, and Millet, B (2011). Major depressive disorder skews the recognition of emotional prosody, *Progress in Neuro-Psychopharmacology and Biological Psychiatry, 35,* 987-996.

[PISANSKI2014] Pisanski, K., Fraccaro, P. J., Tigue, C. C., O'Connor, J. J., Röder, S., Andrews, P. W., Fink, B., DeBruine, L. M., Jones, B. C., & Feinberg, D. R. (2014). Vocal indicators of body size in men and women: A meta-analysis. *Animal Behaviour, 95,* 89–99.

[PISANSKI2019] Pisanski, K., & Bryant, G. A. (2019). The evolution of voice perception . In S. Frühholz & P. Belin (Eds.), *The Oxford Handbook of Voice Perception* (pp. 269–302). Oxford England: Oxford University Press.

[PORGES2001] Porges, S. W. (2001). The polyvagal theory: Phylogenetic substrates of a social nervous system. *International Journal of Psychophysiology, 42*(2), 123–146.

[PORGES2021] Porges, S. W. (2021). *Polyvagal Safety: Attachment, Communication, Self-Regulation* (pp. 73-77). New York: W. W. Norton & Company Inc.

[PORTER1988] Porter, F. L., Porges, S. W., and Marshall, R. E. (1988). Newborn pain cries and vagal tone: parallel changes in response to circumcision. *Child Development, (59),* 495–505.

[PORTFORS2007] Portfors, C. V. (2007). Types and functions of ultrasonic vocalizations in laboratory rats and mice. *Journal of Laboratory Animal Science, 46,* 28–34.

[POSTMA200]. Postma, A. (2000). Detection of errors during speech production: A review of speech monitoring models. *Cognition, 77,* 97–132.

[QATIERI2012] Quatieri, T. F., and Malyska, N. (2012). Vocal-source biomarkers for depression: a link to psychomotor activity. *Proceedings of Interspeech. ICSA,* Portland, USA, pp. 1059–1062.

[RENDALL2005] Rendall, D., Kollias, S., Ney, C., and Lloyd, P. (2005). Pitch (F0) and formant profiles of human vowels and vowel-like baboon grunts: The role of vocalizer body size and voice-acoustic allometry. *The Journal of the Acoustical Society of America, 117,* 944–955.

[SCHERER1986] Scherer, K. R. (1986). Vocal affect expression: A review and a model for future research. *Psychological Bulletin, 99*(2), 143. *https://doi.org/10.1037/0033-2909.99.2.143*

[SCHERER1994] Scherer, K. R. (1994). Affect bursts. In S. H. M. van Goozen, N. E. Van de Poll, & J. A. Sergeant (Eds.), *Emotions: Essays on emotion theory* (pp. 161–193).

[SCHERER2011] Scherer, K. R., Clark-Polner, E., and Mortillaro, M. (2011). In the eye of the beholder? Universality and cultural specificity in the expression and perception of emotion, *International Journal of Psychology, 46(6)*, 401–435.

[SCHERER2013] Scherer, S., Stratou, G., Gratch, J., and Morency, L. P. (2013). Investigating voice quality as a speaker-independent indicator of depression and PTSD. *Interspeech*, 847–851. doi: 10.21437/Interspeech.2013-240.

[SCHERER2016] Scherer, S., Lucas, G. M., Gratch, J., Rizzo, A. S., and Morency, L. P. (2016). Self-reported symptoms of depression and PTSD are associated with reduced vowel space in screening interviews. *IEEE Transactions on Affective Computing, 7(1)*, 59–73.

[SCHLIPF2013] Schlipf, S., Batra, A., Walter, G., Zeep, C., Wildgruber, D., Fallgatter, A. J., and Ethofer, T. (2013). Judgment of emotional information expressed by prosody and semantics in patients with Page 25 of 26 unipolar depression. *Frontiers in Psychology, 4*, 461.

[SIEGMAN1990] Siegman, A. W., Anderson, R. A., and Berger T. (1990). The angry voice: Its effects on the experience of anger and cardiovascular reactivity. *Psychosomatic Medicine, 52(6)*, 631–643. doi: 10.1097/00006842-199011000-00005

[SILVERMAN2010] Silverman, S. E., and Silverman, M. K. (2010). Methods for evaluating near-term suicidal risk using vocal parameters. *Journal of the Acoustical Society of America, 128*, 2259.

[SIMON2017] Simon, D., Becker, M., Mothes-Lasch, M., Miltner, W. H. R., and Starube, T (2017). Loud and angry: Sound intensity modulates amygdala activation to angry voices in social anxiety disorder. *Social Cognitive and Affective Neuroscience, 12(3)*, 409–416.

[SPENCER2016] Spencer, T., Deng, F., El-Feky, M., et al. Tensor tympani muscle. Reference article, Radiopaedia.org (Accessed on 01 Mar 2023)

[STORY1998] Story, B. H., Titze, I. R., and Hoffman, E. A. (1998). Vocal tract area functions for an adult female speaker based on volumetric imaging. *The Journal of the Acoustical Society of America, 104*, 471–487. doi: 10.1121/1.423298

[SUNDBERG2011] Sundberg, J., Patel, S., Bjorkner, E., and Scherer, K. R. (2011). Interdependencies among voice source parameters in emotional speech. *IEEE Transactions on Affective Computing, 2*, 162–174.

[SUNDBERG2013] Sundberg, J., Scherer, R., Hess, M., Müller, F., and Granqvist, S. (2013). Subglottal pressure oscillations accompanying phonation. *Journal of Voice (27)*, 411–421.

[SZABADI1976] Szabadi, E., Bradshaw, C. M., and Besson, J. A. (1976). Elongation of pausetime in speech: A simple, objective measure of motor retardation in depression. *The British Journal of Psychiatry*, 129, 592–597.

[TAYLOR2010] Taylor, A. M., Reby, D., and McComb, K. (2010). Size communication in domestic dog, Canis familiaris, growls. *Animal Behaviour*, 79, 205–210.

[TEASDALE1980] Teasdale, J. D., Fogarty, S. J., and Williams, J. M. G. (1980). Speech rate as a measure of short-term variation in depression. *The British Journal of Social and Clinical Psychology*, 19, 271–278.

[THAYER2009] Thayer, J. F., and Lane, R. D. (2009). Claude Bernard and the heart–brain connection: further elaboration of a model of neurovisceral integration. *Neuroscience & Biobehavioral Reviews, 33*, 81–88. doi: 10.1016/j.neubiorev.2008. 08.004

[TOMATIS1974] Tomatis, A. A. (1974). *Vers l'écoute humaine (2 Vols.)* Paris: Editions E.S.F.

[UEKERMANN2008], Uekermann, J., Abdel-Hamid, M., Lehmkaemper, C., Vollmoeller, W., and Daum, I. (2008). Perception of affective prosody in major depression: A link to executive functions? *Journal of the International Neuropsychological Society, 14*, 552–561.

[URONE2020] Urine, P. P., and Hinrichs, R. (2020). *Physics.* OpenStax: Houston, Book URL: *https://openstax.org/books/physics/pages/1-introduction*

[VANDENBROEK2004]. Van den Broek (2004). Emotional prosody measurement (EPM): a voice-based evaluation method for psychological therapy effectiveness. *Studies in Health Technology and Informatics.*

[VANPUYVELDE2018] Van Puyvelde, M., Neyt, X., McGlone, F., and Pattyn, N. (2018). Voice stress analysis: A new framework for voice and effort in human performance. *Frontiers in Psychology, 20(9)*, *https://www.frontiersin.org/articles/10.3389/fpsyg.2018.01994/full*

[WILEY1978] Wiley, R. H., and Richards, D. B. (1978). Physical constraints on acoustic communication in the atmosphere: implications for the evolution of animal vocalizations. Behav. *Behavioral Ecology and Sociobiology, (3)*, 69–94.

[YAO2016] Yao, X., Chen, B., and Yoshimura, H. (2016). Dynamic features of vocal folds based on speech production model for detection of stressed speech. In *Proceedings of the International Conference Progress in Informatics and Computing (PIC)*, (Shanghai: IEEE), 268–272. doi: 10.1109/PIC.2016.7949508

[YINGTHAWORNSUK2007] Yingthawornsuk, T., Kaymaz-Keskinpala, H., Wilkes, D. M., Shiavi, R. G., and Salomon, R. M. (2007). Direct acoustic feature using iterative EM algorithm and spectral energy for classifying suicidal speech. *Proc. Interspeech* 2007, 766-769, doi: 10.21437/Interspeech.2007-144.

[YOSHIDA1992] Yoshida, Y., Tanaka, Y., Saito, T., Shimazaki, T., and Hirano, M. (1992). Peripheral nervous system in the larynx. *Folia Phoniatrica et Logopaedica* 44, 194–219.

[ZEIPOLLERMANN2002] Zei Pollermann, B., and Archinard, M. (2002). Acoustic patterns of emotions. In E. Keller, G. Bailly, A. Monaghan, J. Terken, & M. Huckvale (Eds.), *Improvements in Speech Synthesis* (pp. 237–245). New York, NY: John Wiley & Sons.

[ZHANG2015]. Zhang, Z. (2015). Regulation of glottal closure and airflow in a three-dimensional phonation model: implications for vocal intensity control. *The Journal of the Acoustical Society of America, 137*, 898–910. doi: 10.1121/1.4906272

[ZHANG2016] Zhang, Z. (2016). Mechanics of human voice production and control, *The Journal of Acoustical Society of America (140)*, 2614.

[ZHOU2004] Zhou, L., Burgoon, J. K., Zhang, D., and Nunamaker, J. F. (2004). Language dominance in interpersonal deception in computer-mediated communication. *Computers in Human Behavior 20*, 381–402.

[ZLOCHOWER1996] Zlochower, A. J., and Cohn, J. F. (1996). Vocal timing in face-to-face interaction of clinically depressed and nondepressed mothers and their 4-month-old infants. *Infant Behavior and Development, 19*, 371–374.

SOCIAL COMMUNICATION: HOW NONVERBAL AND VERBAL ELEMENTS CONVERGE AND ENHANCE OUR COMMUNICATION ABILITIES

What is the difference between describing an internal feeling versus an external object? Why do we often hear adults telling young children to "use their words" when they want the child to explain something upsetting that is happening to them? How does the language we develop through our experiences and various cognitive processes affect how we feel and how we communicate our feelings? The link between language and emotion regulation is a powerful component of communication. As we will see, in this chapter, the ability to understand others' states and to bridge the nonverbal and verbal dimensions of our experiences are key to well-being and optimal communication. Concepts from attachment theory, self-regulation, and feedback responsiveness lay a foundation for understanding how social communication abilities are formed and how this affects our mental health. As we see how our early experiences may influence some of these abilities, this also gives insight into behavior patterns we may deal with as adults and how we may be able to improve our communication abilities.

SOCIAL COMMUNICATION

Social communication is a neuropsychological framework that highlights the socio-cognitive, socio-emotional, and socio-linguistic pillars needed for effective communication. It refers to how humans develop and use appropriate and feedback-responsive verbal and non-verbal elements of communication within a social context [JETHAVA2022; ASHA2021]. It consists of knowing the structural aspects of language like vocabulary and grammar, as well as how to use language to interact with others. An important component of this social communication framework is its emphasis on neuropsychology and its links between language and other cognitive processes like attentional control, information processing, and cognitive flexibility [WISEMAN2020]. These processes, as we have seen in previous chapters, are experience-dependent and therefore influenced significantly by early environments and attachment experiences with caregivers. Earlier researchers such as Vygotsky [VYGOTSKY1934]], Luria [LURIA1966], and more recently Tomas and Vissers [TOMAS2019] highlight the role of neuroscience in understanding the dynamic interplay that occurs between cognitive processes and the development of language, problem-solving, and social-emotional skills. The Social Communication (SoCom) framework discussed below is an integration of many of these theories and current neuropsychological findings that outline the connections between attachment and various realms of social communication including socio-cognitive, socio-emotional, and socio-linguistic skills as well as their interrelated processes like social synchrony, joint attention, and Theory of Mind [JETHAVA2022].

Social communication and executive functioning

As supported by extensive research, socio-cognitive development of executive functioning skills is essential to goal-directed, adaptive behaviors associated with social communication [DIAMOND2013; CARLSON2013; MATTHEWS2018]. Executive functioning supports attentional mechanisms, working memory, cognitive flexibility, and inhibitory control related to self-regulation abilities, which in turn help children learn language by enabling them to stay engaged in and learn from conversations, as well as flexibly apply rules of language needed for constantly changing contexts [JETHAVA2022; HANNO2019]. Moreover, self-regulation abilities have been shown to have an interdependent relationship with language development, where language serves as a tool that can help organize thoughts and plan behavior

[VYGOTSKY1934; HANNO2019]. This interplay occurs in Inner Speech (IS), where children hear and learn from overt speech about their behaviors, such as "I need to wait my turn," and gradually develop this into an internal dialogue that helps direct their behavior and executive functioning skills [VISSERS2020]. Private speech and inner dialogue are mediated by the attachment relationship and are associated with the Theory of Mind (ToM), which is a key to appropriate social communication [HASSANZADEH21018]. We will discuss ToM in an upcoming section.

Social communication and social synchrony

Social synchrony is a foundation for social communication. In Chapter 3, we explored this using the term "biobehavorial synchrony" as a form of attuning and responding to behaviors and internal state changes in a dynamic exchange of hormonal, neurophysiological, and sensory-motor information from one person to another [LECLERE2014; FELDMAN2007]. This type of biobehavioral synchrony can also be referred to as social synchrony. From a neurological perspective, social synchrony is a precursor to the development of the neural empathic network, also called the "neuro-environmental loop of plasticity" [CALLAGHAN2016; YANIV2021]. This neuro-environmental network, which includes the amygdala, insula, temporal pole, and ventromedial prefrontal cortex, underlies emotional functioning, and is developed through interactions with early caregivers [CALLAGHAN2016].

Social Communication and Joint Attention

Social communication is also supported through joint attention. As we saw in Chapter 1, joint attention is another aspect of social communication and is an important milestone that develops in infancy [WISEMAN2020; CLAUSSEN2002]. The first phases of infant-caregiver engagement involve what is called "primary intersubjectivity," which is a person-to-person interaction that involves face-to-face interactions, vocalizations, and eye contact [REDDY2015]. Primary intersubjectivity lays the groundwork for secondary intersubjectivity, where a child and caregiver focus their attention outwards and enter triadic engagement [MOLL2021]. Triadic engagement is the precursor for joint attention, where attention is shared and focused on an external (third) entity rather than on each other [MOLL2021]. Joint attention is seen as a mutually reinforcing feedback mechanism that lays the foundation for the development of neural networks needed for social cognition and language acquisition [MUNDY2017]. Research shows that joint attention and attachment are empirically linked: compared to securely attached children, children with insecure attachment profiles engage in less face-to-face attention and less coordinated joint attention to objects [SCHOLMERICH1997]. A theory proposed by Tomasello and colleagues suggests that this ability to engage in joint attention as it relates to language and social relatedness is due to a uniquely human cognitive feature of shared intentionality [MOLL2021; TOMASELLO2005; 2019; VYGOTSKY2012, p xiii]. This feature enables a child to understand that other humans are intentional agents and emerged from observations that chimpanzees performed equally or better than two-and-a-half-year-old children on cognitive tasks involving spatial memory, rotation of objects, and estimations of quantity but that children clearly outperformed on tasks involving gestures, observational learning, and understanding intentions [VYGOTSKY2012].

Social Communication and Theory of Mind

Theory of Mind (ToM) is another element of social communication and consists of cognitive as well as affective dimensions. First proposed by Woodruff and Premack in the late 1970s, ToM relates to the ability to understand behaviors by creating a mental representation of the self and others [WOODRUFF1978]. This mental representation of the self and others allows a child to understand that another person sees the world differently than how that child sees it. While it eventually applies to others' behavior, ToM development begins with an awareness of one's own internal and external environments [WESTBY2014]. As the caregiver attunes to the infant's gestures, eye gaze, micro-movements, frequencies, and behaviors, this provides live feedback for the infant to develop shared attention and understanding of objects and people's behavior [WESTBY2014]. As the caregiver offers words to describe the infant's internal states and shared objects of attention, this also helps the infant acquire vocabulary. Attunement and ToM (both for the infant and the caregiver) are therefore critical elements for the development of language and communication strategies [VISSERS2016]. Indeed, research shows that the ability of the caregiver to respond to joint attention is associated with the infant's ability to acquire vocabulary [MORALES2000]. Moreover, children whose caregivers ignore their children, react infrequently when their children talk and who use less diverse vocabulary and syntax show challenges in auditory comprehension, smaller vocabularies, and delays in syntactic development [COSTER1993; CULP1991; MCFAYDEN1996].

NONVERBAL AND VERBAL COMPONENTS OF SOCIAL COMMUNICATION

Although caregiver-infant communication is initially primarily based on non-verbal features such as tone of voice, gestures, body postures, and facial expressions, the caregiver's use of words to describe internal states also contributes to the infant's stress modulation and self-regulation abilities [WISEMAN2020]. This process is demonstrated through the concept of "mentalizing," which is the ability to identify and verbalize the mental and emotional states of others and is tied to language development and emotion regulation across the lifespan [BRONSON2000; VALLOTTON2010]. The caregiver's ability to mentalize is also shown to predict the child's later development of empathy and ToM [MEINS2002; TAUMOEPEAU2006].

In terms of neurodevelopment, biobehavioral attunement within caregiver-infant interactions provides the social input needed for an infant to develop skills for appropriate social communication. These include the intersubjectivity of joint attention, mentalizing, and an understanding of others' intentions and perspectives [MUNDY2006; TREVARTHEN2001]. Moreover, children whose caregivers discuss and explain emotions and internal feelings with their children have improved abilities to identify and describe their own experiences and those of others [DUNN1991; SAARNI1997; YEHUDA2005]. Children who can recognize and convey their emotions are also less likely to show signs of depression compared with children who have difficulties in expressing their feelings [RIEFFE2007].

LANGUAGE AS A BRIDGE

Language is a bridge that helps us share our external and internal environments with others. In terms of how it develops, using language to describe concrete objects in our external environment is cognitively less complex because there is an ability to join attention on the object and use sound to help each person's attention converge onto that object. This is the essence of joint attention, which, as we saw in an earlier section, is a foundation of language development. Using language to convey abstract concepts, which include emotions and internal experiences, requires more complex processes. These processes link the subsymbolic (kinesthetic, visceral, and sensory) with the symbolic (verbal and graphical) realm in order to enhance the information we are sharing in our serve-and-return feedback dynamics with others.

We see the trajectory of this process move from general to more complex as children develop emotion categories that first align broadly with their bodily sensations and then move into more fine-grain distinctions [HUPKA1999; RUSSELL1986; SHABLACK2019; WIDEN2013; WIDEN2008). For example, toddlers initially use broad categories of valence to describe their feelings, such as *happy* versus *sad* or *mad*, but begin to incorporate nuances such as *afraid, disgust,* and *surprise* by the time they are five [WIDEN2003]. Moreover, language helps children more accurately identify an emotion from an emotional face, a phenomenon known as "language superiority effect" [RUSSELL1986]. Other research also shows that emotion words affect emotion perception, suggesting that when emotion words are absent, there may be less accuracy of the visual system in recognizing emotion faces [GENDRON2012; LINDQUIST2006].

Using Words to Describe Emotion: Emotional Granularity

As McCrane and Fugate outline in their work on embodied cognition, additional research shows how emotional granularity can enhance emotion regulation and executive function abilities [FUGATE2022]. Emotional granularity, or emotion differentiation, is the ability to recognize fine-grained distinctions between similar feelings such as irritation, impatience, agitation, and annoyance [BARRETT1997; TUGADE2004; FUGATE2018; FUGATE2022]. High emotional granularity is associated with more flexible emotional regulation strategies [BARRETT1997; BODEN2012], as well as fewer maladaptive behaviors such as binge eating [DIXON2014], alcohol abuse [KASHDAN2010], and aggression [POND2012]. In one study, adolescents who were able to make more fine-grained distinctions among negative emotions experienced less intensity of negative feelings and a stronger belief that they were capable of changing their emotions [LENNARZ2018].

Emotional granularity is also associated with mindfulness, which has further correlations with other mental health indicators. The Five Facet Mindfulness Questionnaire (FFMQ) is a widely used measure to assess trait-like mindfulness and involves an assessment of verbal emotional granularity. One of the five facets is the describing facet, which reports on an individual's ability to find words to describe their feelings, beliefs, opinions, and expectations [BAER 2006; FUGATE2022]. Studies have shown that individuals who score higher on the describing facet self-report greater attention to and clarity of emotions and lower symptoms of alexithymia (which we will cover in an upcoming section) [BAER2006]. The FFMQ also reveals consistent associations of higher scores on the describing facet corresponding to lower symptoms of anxiety, depression, and related disorders, as well as higher quality of life [CARPENTER2019; MATTES2019; BODEN2015]. Of all the facets of the FFMQ, the described facet shows the strongest connection to social outcomes, as suggested by a meta-analysis [MATTES2019].

Alexithymia and Challenges in Describing Emotions

On the other side of the spectrum, an inability to describe emotions and internal states has strong relationships with various mental health challenges. One field of exploration into this relates to alexithymia. The term alexithymia was first proposed in the 1970s by Peter Sifneos, a psychiatrist, professor, and researcher working with patients experiencing psychosomatic illnesses and other mental health disorders. He used the term alexithymia to describe a cluster of symptoms related to an inability to identify and label emotional feeling states [NEMIAH1976; NEMIAH1970]. Since then, the alexithymia construct has been integrated into many different streams of mental health research, including post-traumatic stress, anxiety, and depression. Research over the past couple of decades has also provided enough empirical support for the validity of the alexithymia construct and the creation of a reliable and valid measurement tool, The Toronto Alexithymia Scale (TAS) [TAYLOR2000]. Key features of the construct include a diminished ability to identify and describe feeling states and difficulty distinguishing between specific feelings and bodily sensations associated with emotional arousal [TAYLOR2000]. According to some theoretical models for understanding alexithymia, the limited ability to verbally express feelings is related to an impairment in cognitive processing, regulation, and mental representations of emotions [TAYLOR2000; TAYLOR1991; SAMUR2018]. This model is based on the idea that emotion regulation involves three interrelated systems: neurophysiological, motor-expressive, and cognitive-experiential [TAYLOR2000].

An added challenge for individuals with high levels of alexithymia is that not only do they have difficulties in reflecting on and regulating their emotions, but they also have a hard time communicating their distress and need for help or comfort from others [TAYLOR2000].

The lack of emotion-sharing then continues to lead to a lack of feedback and attunement from others, which creates further deficits in the alexithymic individual's ability to identify their emotions [TAYLOR2000]. The connection between alexithymia and emotion regulation has received empirical support through studies using the Affect Regulation Scale (ARS). This scale evaluates the various coping strategies people use to manage distressing emotions [TAYLOR2000]. In a study on psychiatric outpatients, alexithymia was positively associated with maladaptive emotion regulation strategies, such as binging on food [TAYLOR2000; RICE2022]. Higher levels of alexithymia were also associated with fewer adaptive strategies such as trying to understand or talking about distressing emotions with a caring other [TAYLOR2000]. A study on male parolees using the ARS also found associations between alexithymia and maladaptive emotion regulation behaviors such as sexual and aggressive behavior, drinking alcohol, and reckless activities [TAYLOR2000; BECKENDAM1977]. Other studies have shown a high prevalence of alexithymia among male prisoners, with rates ranging between 31% and 47%, almost three times higher than is estimated in general populations [HEMMING2021; ZIMMERMAN2006; CHEN2017] and that high prevalence of alexithymia among prisoners is related to their level of education, adverse childhood experiences and symptoms of negative emotions [CHEN2017]. Male adolescent offenders have also been reported to score high on alexithymia and show a higher prevalence of coming from disrupted family structures than control groups [ZIMMERMAN2006].

Cognitive, Emotional, and Linguistic Aspects of Alexithymia

Our emotion regulation and language abilities are built on serve-and-return exchanges with others. One model proposed by Land and Schwartz reflects a developmental process of how bodily sensations related to emotions gradually increase in nuance and complexity and become associated with and symbolized in words [LANE1987]. This model has been further refined into the "multiple code theory," which proposes that nonverbal schemas develop first and include subsymbolic processes (sensory, visceral, and kinesthetic sensations) combined with symbolic imagery and are later developed into verbal emotion schemas [TAYLOR2000; BUCCI1997]. These verbal and nonverbal schemas are connected via referential links, meaning that one or more reference points need to connect the feelings with an image or symbol [BUCCI1997A]. These referential links are the most distant for sensory experiences and autonomic arousal, which means they may need a specific image within the nonverbal domain before they can be linked with words from the verbal domain [BUCCI1997; SAMUR2018]. Because of this, the issue with alexithymia may be that a person not only lacks words to describe their emotions but also verbal and nonverbal symbols to link with their internal states. This means that as a physiological activation occurs during emotional arousal, it does not activate an associated cognitive process, which can lead to prolonged, repetitive, or more severe levels of dysregulation [BUCCI1997].

In line with the multiple code theory, earlier theories proposed that the impaired ability to verbally express feelings is tied to impaired abilities to mentally represent and cognitively process emotions [TAYLOR1991; SAMUR2018]. To understand this cognitive-emotional-communication connection even further, we can look at how people link words to their emotions. In order to know a word that links to something, there must be a cognitive representation of this that contains information about pronunciation, syntax, meaning, and how a word has individual connotations [AITCHISON2012]. Our unique mental processes interweave with our unique individual experiences of each moment to form concepts and associate them with words that symbolize those concepts [LOBNER2011]. For concrete objects in our external environment, this process has less complexity because the image already has sensory input that links it with image-based processing. Emotions, on the other hand, do not have this direct link to a symbol or image. As we have seen in previous chapters, emotions, and affective states are a combination of processes that involve our evaluations of stimuli and perceived ability to cope, as well as attentional mechanisms related to our internal state and anticipatory adjustments. In that sense, emotions are abstractions of scenes, objects, and people and how they come together into an evaluation and corresponding internal state fluctuation [BUCCI1997]. As multiple code theory suggests, these abstractions are emotional concepts and are represented at symbolic and/or subsymbolic levels. The subsymbolic level involves the visceral, sensory, and kinesthetic sensations that occur in a person's internal state during their experiences. The symbolic realm includes images and linguistic information. As a person interacts with a scene (which includes their assessment of a situation, object, or person) and experiences an internal state fluctuation, the emotion is initially processed at the subsymbolic level [BUCCI1997]. Shortly after, their attention then goes to the symbolic level, where images and verbal encodings are linked with the internal world [BUCCI1997]. People with high levels of alexithymia seem to have challenges within this process of linking the subsymbolic with the symbolic realms, translating those internal and emotional experiences into words. Because of this, the internal state fluctuations and related emotional arousal levels remain at the subsymbolic (visceral, sensory, and kinesthetic sensation) level [BUCCI1997; SAMUR2018]. With their attention not being directed to cognitive processes, a person may not be able to access regulatory strategies to regulate, differentiate, and understand these internal processes, as well as communicate them outwardly into symbols and language that another person could understand [BUCCI1997; SAMUR2018].

Research that explores how conditions such as alexithymia affect language can help us explore various psychological dimensions of language. For example, a variety of studies have found that people with high alexithymia (HA) use fewer emotional words in their speech and have less complex emotional vocabulary [JELINEK2010; LUMINET2004; PAEZ1999; ROEDEMA1999; TULL2005; VANHEULE2011; WOTSCHACK2013]. Moreover, high levels of alexithymia have also been associated with a withdrawn communication style and a tendency to not open up to others [KREITLER2002; WAGNER2008].

While the use of words and verbal expression is clearly important for emotion regulation and social communication, both the verbal and nonverbal components of emotional cues are important for social communication. In the next section, we will look at how emotional cues are prioritized by brain networks and nervous system mechanisms for faster processing. Understanding this can also help us understand how subliminal and subconscious processes related specifically to emotional cues contribute to our communication behaviors and patterns.

PRIORITIZATION OF EMOTIONAL CUES IN VERBAL AND NONVERBAL COMMUNICATION

A person's emotional state is an important factor in whether they are safe to approach and how they may interact with others. Various neural systems reflect this prioritization and are devoted to processing emotional input more quickly than other types of information. For example, face perception appears to rely on a fast neural pathway to analyze emotional expressions quickly and grossly, while a slower pathway is used for identifying and recognizing finer details as well as precise identity features [NOESSELT2002; POURTOIS2004; WEST2011]. This aligns with findings that low-spatial frequency is enough to convey coarse facial expressions, while fine-grained details of a face require more time-consuming, high spatial frequencies [COSTEN1996; LIU2000]. For example, emotional expressions in faces can be conveyed by low spatial frequency cues of two to eight cycles/face—coarseness of input that can be processed from faces in the periphery, at a distance, or in motion [LIVINGSTONE1988; MERIGAN1993]. Researchers suggest that faster processing of coarse emotional input offers an evolutionary advantage for subconsciously assessing input that is time-sensitive and potentially critical for survival and communication [VUILLEUMIER2003; JOHNSON2005].

Research reveals this in additional studies where emotional faces are more readily detected than neutral faces [EASTWOOD2001; FOX2002], and people's attention is more easily drawn to emotional stimuli than neutral stimuli [ANDERSON2005; PHELPS2005; VUILLEUMIER2005].

Neural circuitry devoted to faster processing from coarse emotional cues has evolutionary roots in our detection of threats. For example, determining the general outline, widening, and gaze direction of eyes is visible at low-spatial frequency [WHALEN2004]. These are important cues to understanding a person's internal state and intentions, as well as what dangers they may be perceiving in their environment that could harm them or whether they perceive us as a threat and may move to attack. Because a newborn infant's vision is still in development, the ability of a caregiver to convey emotional expressions using low-frequency cues allow these cues to be perceived by the infant, who still lacks a mature visual cortex [JOHNSON2005]. This contrasts with the high spatial frequency cues (8–16 cycles/face) needed for fine-grained and accurate face identification [FIORENTINI1983; LIU2000]. We see from these examples that the brain-body system has established a form of prioritization for emotional cues—particularly at the coarse, low-spatial frequency level. An understanding of this prioritization of emotional cues can help deepen our understanding of communication patterns, as they reveal how quickly and unconsciously our senses may be reacting to the visual and auditory input it is receiving from others.

This prioritization of emotional cues is also seen in brain structures, and in particular the amygdala, which is thought to play a key role in assessing the salience of emotional stimuli [LEDOUX2000; SANDER2003A; PHELPS2005]. Salience refers to an evaluation of an input's significance: when something is salient, it means it is noticeable in terms of its importance to us. Studies suggest that coarse visual information from emotional cues (e.g., eyes widening) [WHALEN2004] is processed quickly by the amygdala before being sent to the visual cortex for enhanced processing of information [VUILLEUMIER2003; 2005]. The amygdala is modulated by coarse low-spatial frequency cues [LIEBENTHAL2016] and receives major inputs with coarse resolution through a retinal-superior colliculus-pulvinar subcortical pathway [SCHILLER1979; LIVINGSTONE1988; MERIGAN1993]. This pathway allows for faster processing of fear-related and emotion-related [ZALD2003] data by bypassing the slower cortical route of the ventral-visual pathway [LEDOUX1996; MORRIS1999; DEGELDER200]. As we see from this, emotional cues, and in particular fear-related cues, are processed more quickly than other types of information.

Lateralization

Research suggests that these slower versus faster processing routes also emerge in terms of the left and right hemispheres playing different roles in verbal and nonverbal emotion perception. Lateralization is a term used to describe different, specialized functions of the left and right hemispheres of the brain. The amygdala is one area of the brain where we see some of this lateralization. For example, in terms of face processing, responses are shorter, and adaptation is faster in the right amygdala compared to the left [WRIGHT2001; GLASCHER2004; COSTAFREDA2008; SERGERIE2008]. The right amygdala is also predominantly activated by subliminal emotional stimuli compared to the left [MORRIS1998; GLASCHER2003; PEGNA2005]. The amygdala also lateralizes its processing of language, with activation occurring predominantly in the left amygdala when emotional information is conveyed exclusively through language [PHELPS2001; OLSSON2004]. Researchers suggest that the right amygdala serves primarily as an emotion detector, responding quickly and subconsciously via subcortical routes (namely the superior colliculus-pulvinar-amygdala pathway) [LEDOUX1984; MORRIS1999]. The left amygdala appears to respond via an indirect, cortical route, making its responses slower in order to evaluate the significance of emotional stimuli [VUILLEUMIER2003; WINSTON2003]. It is important to note, however, that although these studies highlight the possibility of amygdalar processing and lateralization, other findings also suggest that there may be multiple parallel routes for prioritizing and processing emotional stimuli that are in addition to or do not involve the amygdala [ADOLPHS2005; TSUCHIYA2009; LIEBENTHAL2016].

Faster Processing of Nonverbal Emotional Vocalizations

Because vocalizations contain both verbal and nonverbal components, clinicians and researchers have also looked at how the brain processes nonverbal emotional vocalizations. Nonverbal emotional vocalizations communicate meaning without using words, such as laughing and crying [SAMUR2018]. Similar to the faster processing and prioritized routes for emotional faces, emotional voices also appear to have a perceptual advantage compared with neutral nonspeech vocalizations [ARMONY2007]. Emotional nonverbal vocalizations such as screams, cries, or laughs are related to heightened activity in the amygdala and the auditory superior temporal cortex [PHILLIPS1998; MORRIS1999; FECTEAU2007], regardless of attentional state [SANDER2001]. Further research suggests that the amygdala may be particularly sensitive to short, nonverbal emotional vocalizations and that this may be because the short bursts of this information can be more quickly processed than the longer time scale needed for speech prosody [SANDER2005; BACH2008; FRUHHOLZ2012]. Similar to the findings on visual emotional cues that point to the amygdala as an emotional intensity detector, some findings on rising intensity in voices also show a higher activation in the right amygdala [BACH2008].

Perception of Emotional Written Words

As we have seen from the concept of emotional granularity, words can add dimensions that help refine and nuance the emotional state being conveyed. Two primary dimensions that emerge in research on emotional content of written words are valence and arousal [BRADLEY1999; WARRINER2013]. Valence refers to the positive or negative emotional association, while arousal refers to salience or significance and the associated nervous system mechanisms that occur due to that salience. For example, something highly salient will draw attention (versus not being noticed) and will therefore activate blood flow and brain activity accordingly. The salience of a stimulus combined with valence will influence whether a person not only pays attention to and prioritizes their attention to that stimulus but also whether they will report it as pleasing or aversive. Some studies show differentiation in the amygdala and other brain areas in response to word arousal and word valence [LEWIS2007; POSNER2009; COLLIBAZZI2010]. However, language stimuli are generally less likely to activate the amygdala, particularly in the right hemisphere [ANDERSON2001; PHELPS2001; OLSSON2004; GOLDSTEIN2007; COSTAFREDA2008]. Researchers suggest that this weak activity in the amygdala in response to words may be because the amygdala is less involved in language processing or even that the prefrontal cortex may inhibit amygdala activity during this process [BECHARA1995; ROSENKRANZ2003; PEZAWAS2005; BLAIR2007]. Moreover, the subjective relevance of words may result in a large diversity of responses across populations. For example, in studies on people with posttraumatic stress disorder (PTSD), the left amygdala showed high levels of activation and abnormal patterns of sensitization and habituation compared to controls for trauma-related negative words but not for panic-related or neutral words [PROTOPOPESCU2005].

Extensive research has shown that emotionally arousing words (positive and negative) are processed more quickly and activate differential brain responses than neutral words [KISSLER2006; THOMAS2007; HERBERT2008;

SCHACHT2009; SCOTT2009; CITRON2011]. Although it is not clear whether there is a fast subcortical route for the subliminal processing of emotional words, research does suggest that the left amygdala has a lateralized dominance for language compared to the right amygdala, which aligns with the general dominance of the entire left hemisphere for language [LIEBENTHAL2014; NAKIC2006]. This left and right-lateralized activity when it comes to emotion processing, reflects the right-brain regulation processes that occur through nonverbal communication, particularly between infants and caregivers [SCHORE2008]. It also highlights how we can further attempt to understand the link between the subsymbolic realm of visceral, sensory, and kinesthetic senses with symbolic and verbal processes. It aligns with sayings we may have heard about helping kids explain how they are feeling when we say "use your words," or "name it to tame it" [SIEGEL2012]. The studies on alexithymia and emotion granularity further validate the importance of being able to refine and supplement our nonverbal signals with words and language.

Perception of Emotional Spoken Words

In addition to emotional written words, emotional spoken words also reveal a prioritization of processing within the brain. In contrast to written words, however, spoken words are supplemented by nonverbal information coming from voice frequencies and their relationship to internal physiological states [KOTZ2007; PELL2011]. Spoken language contains a variety of spectrotemporal properties. The concept of spectrotemporal modulation is important in our understanding of communication because it underlies the type of signals that are processed by the brain.[1] Phonemic cues (phonemes[2]) and prosodic cues are spectrotemporal properties of speech. Phonemic cues are sounds that consist of fast spectral changes occurring within 50 ms time segments of speech, meaning every 50 ms, there is a change of frequency on the sound

---

[1] Spectrotemporal represents an interaction between wavelengths and time, and usually refers to auditory processes. [GAUCHER2013] This is in comparison to spatiotemporal, which generally refers to visual processes in which a stimulus is processed in the brain in terms of its spatial location and time. If there are issues with auditory processing, this may have an effect on how a person may respond to the vocal cues they are receiving. For example, if their processing speed is slow, then it can be difficult for them to follow someone's speech because they are still processing a sound made earlier, while the person continues to say words, creating a type of backlog and challenge in understanding.

[2] Phonemes are units of sounds that make up human speech.

spectrum [LIEBENTHAL2016]. Prosodic cues take longer to produce because they are combinations of sounds that form together into patterns that convey emotion and are contained in syllables and suprasegmental units[3] [LIEBENTHAL2016]. Emotional speech consists of both prosodic and phonemic elements, which convey sound frequencies that are given a processing advantage such as higher intelligibility in environments with background noise [NYGAARD2008; GORDON2011; DUPUIS2014]. Emotional speech also undergoes a more efficient processing that allows for faster repetition when the prosody of voice is congruent with the emotional words being spoken [NYGAARD2008; GORDON2011; DUPUIS2014]. Research points to the idea that nonverbal emotional vocalizations are processed quickly via subcortical routes similar to emotional cues from faces, emotional prosody can only be conveyed over longer time scales, and therefore likely have more indirect routes from the auditory to the association cortices [LIEBENTHAL2016]. This is also helpful for us to understand because prosodic cues do not use a fast route to the amygdala; there may be room for humans to exercise cortical resources for modulating the perception, interpretation, and expression of prosodic information in the voice.

Similar to written words, the concept of lateralization comes up again in relation to the perception of spoken words. Research suggests a higher sensitivity in the right hemisphere to spectral cues that emerge over relatively longer time scales, such as prosodic cues, and a higher sensitivity in the left hemisphere to fast and brief spectral changes (such as phonemic cues) [ZATORRE2001; BOEMIO2005; POEPPEL2008]. These differences are also commonly found in fMRI studies that reveal a right hemisphere dominance for perceiving emotional prosody and a left hemisphere dominance for comprehending speech [MITCHELL2003; GRANDJEAN2005]. One proposed theory for these differences relates to the innate properties of the neurons in the left hemisphere that make them more predisposed to processing short time scales compared with the oscillatory properties of the right hemisphere's neurons [GIRAUD2007; GIRAUD2012]. Other proposed explanations for the hemispheric differences in processing linguistic versus nonlinguistic cues relate to the differences in higher-order areas that feed into the auditory cortex [LIEBENTHAL2016]. In alignment with research on alexithymia, these hemispheric differences are particularly important for our understanding

---

[3] Suprasegmental are elements of speech that are above the smaller units of phonemes, consonants, and vowels [KAMILOGLU2021].

of communication patterns and their connection to mental health, emotion regulation, and social dynamics.

As a brief review from Chapter 6, the voice has particular importance and ability to convey internal state information because the frequencies can reach another person from a distance without the proximity needed for accurate facial cue detection [LIEBENTHAL2016]. The voice is also inextricably linked and modulated by a person's physiological state, including breathing patterns, heart rate, and muscle tension, which makes it an important medium for transmitting and detecting information quickly and without the added cortical processes needed for words and language. Two particular nonverbal features help convey some of this emotional and internal state information: prosody and quality of nonspeech vocalization. Prosody, as mentioned earlier in this chapter and in Chapter 6, refers to speech intonations that include pitch, loudness, and rhythm. Prosodic features are suprasegmental, meaning they are a combination of multiple segments of speech and therefore only emerge relatively slowly compared to short, abrupt bursts of nonspeech vocalizations [PELL2015]. Non-speech vocalizations contain abrupt spectral changes that can quickly and potently convey emotional information, such as fear and disgust [BANSE1996; SCOT1997]. For example, rising sound intensity is theorized to be a primal auditory warning cue [NEUHOFF1998] and leads to higher activation in the right amygdala compared to a decline in sound intensity [BACH2008]. We can see from various studies that short nonspeech vocalizations are a fast way to convey important emotional cues. For example, research reveals that the amygdala is particularly activated by short, nonverbal emotional vocalizations [SANDER2003; FECTEAU2007; FRUHHOLZ2014]. The amygdala also appears to have particularly high activity when processing emotional vocalizations [SANDER2005; BACH2008; FRUHHOLZ2012]. This type of amygdala activity in relation to emotional vocalizations parallels what we see in terms of the fast subliminal processing of visual input from emotional faces [SANDER2003A].

SUMMARY

As we see from the above studies, the brain-body system uses a variety of strategies to process emotional information. Put together, we see that emotional cues, compared with neutral ones, are processed differently than other stimuli. Our communication behaviors and patterns are influenced by our emotional states, expressions, and language in ways that are not necessarily conscious of us but are being prioritized and responded to by our senses and nervous system. This makes the topic of emotions and emotion regulation central to any discussion of communication. The more we can learn how they are formed, expressed, detected, and processed, the more we can explore how to improve our skills in matching what we are saying with what we are feeling and intending. In the next chapter, we will look at how developmental processes of maturity and systems dynamics play a role in the interaction of emotion regulation and communication.

REFERENCES

[ADOLPHS2005] Adolphs, R., Tranel, D., and Buchanan, T. W. (2005). Amygdala damage impairs emotional memory for gist but not details of complex stimuli. *Nature Neuroscience*, 8, 512–518. doi: 10.1038/nn

[AITCHISON2012] Aitchison, J. (2012). *Words in the Mind: An Introduction to the Mental Lexicon*. West Sussex: John Wiley & Sons.

[ANDERSON2001] Anderson, A. K., and Phelps, E. A. (2001). Lesions of the human amygdala impair enhanced

[ANDERSON2005] Anderson, A. K. (2005). Affective influences on the attentional dynamics supporting awareness. *The Journal of Experimental Psychology: General, 134*, 258–281. doi: 10.1037/0096-3445.134.2.258

[ARMONY2007] Armony, J. L., Chochol, C., Fecteau, S., and Belin, P. (2007). Laugh (or cry) and you will be remembered: influence of emotional expression on memory for vocalizations. *Psychological Science, 18*, 1027–1029. doi: 10.1111/j.1467-9280.2007.02019.x

[ASHA2021] American Speech-Language-Hearing Association. *Social Communication [Internet]*. Rockville, ML: ASHA (1997–2022). (accessed December 2, 2021).

[BACH2008] Bach, D. R., Schächinger, H., Neuhoff, J. G., Esposito, F., Di Salle, F., Lehmann, C., et al. (2008). Rising sound intensity: an intrinsic warning cue activating the amygdala. *Cerebral Cortex*, 18, 145–150. doi: 10.1093/cercor/bhm040

[BAER2006] Baer, R. A., Smith, G. T., Hopkins, J., Krietemeyer, J., and Toney, L. (2006). Using self-report assessment methods to explore facets of mindfulness. *Assessment, 13(1)*, 27–45.

[BANSE1996] Banse, R., and Scherer, K. R. (1996). Acoustic profiles in vocal emotion expression. *Journal of Personality and Social Psychology*, 70, 614–636. doi: 10.1037/0022-3514.70.3.614

[BARRETT1997] Barrett, L. F. (1997). The relationship among momentary emotional experiences, personality descriptions, and retrospective ratings of emotion. *Personality and Social Psychology Bulletin, 23*, 1100–1110.

[BECHARA1995] Bechara, A., Tranel, D., Damasio, H., Adolphs, R., Rockland, C., and Damasio, A. R. (1995). Double dissociation of conditioning and declarative knowledge relative to the amygdala and hippocampus in humans. *Science,* 269, 1115–1118. doi: 10.1126/science.7652558

[BECKENDAM1977] Beckendam C. (1977). Dimensions of emotional intelligence: attachment, affect regulation, alexithymia and empathy. Doctoral Dissertation, The Fielding Institute, SantaBarbara, CA.

[BLAIR2007] Blair, K. S., Smith, B. W., Mitchell, D. G., Morton, J., Vythilingam, M., Pessoa, L., et al. (2007). Modulation of emotion by cognition and cognition by emotion. *Neuroimage, 35*, 430–440. doi: 10.1016/j.neuroimage.2006.11.048

[BODEN2012] Boden, M. T., & Berenbaum, H. (2012). Facets of emotional clarity and suspiciousness. *Personality and Individual Differences, 53(4)*, 426–430.

[BODEN2015] Boden, M. T., Irons, J. G., Feldner, M. T., Bujarski, S., and Bonn-Miller, M. O. (2015). An investigation of relations among quality of life and individual facets of emotional awareness and mindfulness. *Mindfulness, 6(4)*, 700–707.

[BOEMIO2005] Boemio, A., Fromm, S., Braun, A., and Poeppel, D. (2005). Hierarchical and asymmetric temporal sensitivity in human auditory cortices. *Nature Neuroscience, 8*, 389–395. doi: 10.1038/nn1409

[BRADLEY1999] Bradley, M. M., and Lang, P. J. (1999). *Affective Norms for English Words (ANEW): Instruction Manual and Affective Ratings.* Gainesville, FL: NIMH Center for Emotion and Attention, University of Florida.

[BRONSON2000] Bronson, M. B. (2000) Recognizing and supporting the development of self-regulation in young children. *Young Child.* (55) 32–X.

[BUCCI1997] Bucci, W. (1997). Psychoanalysis and Cognitive Science: A Multiple Code Theory. New York: Guilford Press.

[BUCCI1997A] Bucci, W. (1997). Symptoms and symbols: a multiple code theory of somatization. *Psycho-analytic Inquiry, (17)*, 151–72.24.

[CALLAGHAN2016] Callaghan, B. L., and Tottenham, N. (2016). The neuro-environmental loop of plasticity: A cross-species analysis of parental effects on emotion circuitry development following typical and adverse caregiving. *Neuropsychopharmacology, (41)*, 163–76. 10.1038/npp.2015.204

[CARLSON2013] Carlson, S. M., Zelazo, P. D., and Faja, S. (2013). Executive function. In: Zelazo, P.D. (Ed.) *The Oxford Handbook of Developmental Psychology* (pp. 706–43, Vol. 1), New York, NY: Oxford University Press.

[CARPENTER2019] Carpenter, J. K., Conroy, K., Gomez, A. F., Curren, L. C., aand Hofmann, S. G. (2019). The relationship between trait mindfulness and affective symptoms: A meta-analysis of the Five Facet Mindfulness Questionnaire (FFMQ). *Clinical Psychology Review, 74,* Article 101785. *https://doi.org /10.1016/j.cpr.2019.101785*

[CHEN2017] Chen, L., Xu, L., You, W., Zhang, X., and Ling, N. (2017). Prevalence and associated factors of alexithymia among adult prisoners in China: a cross-sectional study. *BMC Psychiatry, 17,* 287. doi: 10.1186/s12888-017-1443-7

[CITRON2011] Citron, F. M., Oberecker, R., Friederici, A. D., and Mueller, J. L. (2011). Mass counts: ERP correlates of non-adjacent dependency learning under different exposure conditions. *Neuroscience Letters, 487,* 282–286. doi: 10.1016/j.neulet.2010.10.038

[CLAUSSEN2002] Claussen, A. H., Mundy, P. C., Mallik, S. A., and Willoughby, J. C. (2002). Joint attention and disorganized attachment status in infants at risk. *Development and Psychopathology, (14),* 279–291. 10.1017/s0954579402002055

[COLIBAZZI2010] Colibazzi, T., Posner, J., Wang, Z., Gorman, D., Gerber, A., Yu, S., et al. (2010). Neural systems subserving valence and arousal during the experience of induced emotions. *Emotion, 10,* 377–389. doi: 10.1037/a0018484

[COSTAFREDA2008] Costafreda, S. G., Brammer, M. J., David, A. S., and Fu, C. H. (2008). Predictors of amygdala activation during the processing of emotional stimuli: a meta-analysis of 385 PET and fMRI studies. *Brain Research Reviews, 58,* 57–70. doi: 10.1016/j.brainresrev.2007.10.012

[COSTEN1996] Costen, N. P., Parker, D. M., and Craw, I. (1996). Effects of high-pass and low-pass spatial filtering on face identification. *Perception & Psychophysics, 58,* 602–612. doi: 10.3758/BF03213093

[COSTER1993] Coster, W., and Cicchetti, D. (1993) Research on the communicative development of maltreated children: Clinical implications. *Top Languages Discord Servers, (13)*, 25–38. 10.1097/00011363-199308000-00007

[CULP1991] Culp, R. E., Watkins, R. V., Lawrence, H., Letts, D., Kelly, D. J., and Rice, M. L. (1991). Maltreated children's language and speech development: abused, neglected, and abused and neglected. *First Language, (11)*, 377–389.

[DIAMOND2013] Diamond, A. (2013). Executive functions. *Annual Review of Psychology, 64*, 135–168.

[DIXON2014] Dixon-Gordon, K. L., Chapman, A. L., Weiss, N. H., and Rosenthal, M. Z. (2014). A preliminary examination of the role of emotion differentiation in the relationship between borderline personality and urges for maladaptive behaviors. *Journal of Psychopathology and Behavioral Assessment, 36(4)*, 616–625.

[DUNN1991] Dunn, J., Brown, J., Slomkowski, C., Tesla, C., & Youngblade, L. M. (1991). Young children's understanding of other people's feelings and beliefs: Individual differences and their antecedents. *Child Development, 62*, 1352–1366.

[DUPUIS2014] Dupuis, K., and Pichora-Fuller, M. K. (2014). Intelligibility of emotional speech in younger and older adults. *Ear Hearing, 35*, 695–707.

[EASTWOOD2001] Eastwood, J. D., Smilek, D., and Merikle, P. M. (2001). Differential attentional guidance by unattended faces expressing positive and negative emotion. *Perception & Psychophysics, 63*, 1004–1013. doi: 10.3758/BF03194519

[FECTEAU2007] Fecteau, S., Belin, P., Joanette, Y., and Armony, J. L. (2007). Amygdala responses to nonlinguistic emotional vocalizations. *Neuroimage, 36*, 480–487. doi: 10.1016/j.neuroimage.2007.02.043

[FELDMAN2007] Feldman, R. (2007). Parent–infant synchrony: biological foundations and developmental outcomes. *Current Directions in Psychological Science, (16)*, 340–345. 10.1111/j.1467-8721.2007.00532

[FIORENTINI1983] Fiorentini, A., Maffei, L., and Sandini, G. (1983). The role of high spatial frequencies in face perception. *Perception, 12*, 195–201. doi: 10.1068/p120195

[FLINKER 2019] Flinker, A., Doyle, W. K., Mehta, A. D., et al. (2019). Spectrotemporal modulation provides a unifying framework for auditory cortical asymmetries. *Nature Human Behaviour, 3*, 393–405.

[FOX2002] Fox, E. (2002). Processing emotional facial expressions: the role of anxiety and awareness. *Cognitive, Affective, & Behavioral Neuroscience, 2*, 52–63. doi: 10.3758/CABN.2.1.52

[FRUHHOLZ2012] Frühholz, S., Ceravolo, L., and Grandjean, D. (2012). Specific brain networks during explicit and implicit decoding of emotional prosody. *Cerebral Cortex, 22*, 1107–1117. doi: 10.1093/cercor/bhr184

[FRUHHOLZ2014] Frühholz, S., Trost, W., and Grandjean, D. (2014). The role of the medial temporal limbic system in processing emotions in voice and music. *Progress in Neurobiology, 123*, 1–17. doi: 10.1016/j.pneurobio.2014.09.003

[FUGATE2018] Fugate, J. M. B., Macrine, S. L., and Cipriano, C. (2018). The role of embodied cognition for transforming learning. *International Journal of School & Educational Psychology, 7(4)*, 274–288.

[FUGATE2022] Fugate, J. M. B., and Wilson-Mendenhall, C. (2022). Embodied emotion, emotional granularity, and mindfulness: improved learning in the classroom. In *Movement Matters: How Embodied Cognition Informs Teaching and Learning.* Editors S. L. Macrine and J. M. B. Fugate. Cambridge, MA: MIT Press, pp. 291-306.

[GAUCHER2013] Gaucher, Q., Huetz, C., Gourévitch, B., Laudanski, J., Occelli, F., and Edeline, J. M. (2013). How do auditory cortex neurons represent communication sounds?, *Hearing Research, (305)*: 102–112.

[GENDRON2012] Gendron, M., Lindquist, K. A., Barsalou, L., and Barrett, L. F. (2012). Emotion words shape emotion percepts. *Emotion, 12(2)*, 314–325.

[GIRAUD2007] Giraud, A. L., Kleinschmidt, A., Poeppel, D., Lund, T. E., Frackowiak, R. S., and Laufs, H. (2007). Endogenous cortical rhythms determine cerebral specialization for speech perception and production. *Neuron, 56*, 1127–1134. doi: 10.1016/j.neuron.2007.09.038

[GIRAUD2012] Giraud, A. L., and Poeppel, D. (2012). Cortical oscillations and speech processing: emerging computational principles and operations. *Nature Neuroscience, 15*, 511–517. doi: 10.1038/nn.3063

[GLASCHER2004] Gläscher, J., Tuscher, O., Weiller, C., and Buchel, C. (2004). Elevated responses to constant facial emotions in different faces in the human amygdala: an fMRI study of facial identity and expression. *BMC Neuroscience, 5,* 45. doi: 10.1186/1471-2202-5-45

[GOLDSTEIN2007] Goldstein, M., Brendel, G., Tuescher, O., Pan, H., Epstein, J., Beutel, M., et al. (2007). Neural substrates of the interaction of emotional stimulus processing and motor inhibitory control: An emotional linguistic go/no-go fMRI study. *Neuroimage, 36,* 1026–1040. doi: 10.1016/j.neuroimage.2007.01.056

[GORDON2011] Gordon, M. S., and Hibberts, M. (2011). Audiovisual speech from emotionally expressive and lateralized faces. *Quarterly Journal of Experimental Psychology,* 64, 730–750. doi: 10.1080/17470218.2010.516835

[GRANDJEAN2005] Grandjean, D., Sander, D., Pourtois, G., Schwartz, S., Seghier, M. L., Scherer, K. R., et al. (2005). The voices of wrath: brain responses to angry prosody in meaningless speech. *Nature Neuroscience,* 8, 145–146. Doi: 10.1038/nn1392

[HANNO2019] Hanno, E., and Surrain, S. (2019). The direct and indirect relations between self-regulation and language development among monolinguals and dual language learners. *Clinical Child and Family Psychology Review,* (22), 75–79.

[HASSANZADEH21018]. Hassanzadeh, S., and Amraei, K.(2018). The study of mediating role of private speech in conceptual model of relationship between language development, secure attachment and behavioral self-regulation. *Journal of Applied Psychology,* (8), 37–50.

[HEMMING2021] Hemming, L., Shaw, J., Haddock, G., Carter, L. A., and Pratt D. (2021). A cross-sectional study investigating the relationship between alexithymia and suicide, violence, and dual harm in male prisoners. *Frontiers in Psychiatry, 12,* 670863. *https://doi.org/10.3389/fpsyt.2021.670863.*

[HERBERT2008] Herbert, C., Junghofer, M., and Kissler, J. (2008). Event related potentials to emotional adjectives during reading. *Psychophysiology, 45,* 487–498. doi: 10.1111/j.1469-8986.2007.00638.x

[HUPKA1999] Hupka, R. B., Lenton, A. P., and Hutchison, K. A. (1999). Universal development of emotion categories in natural language. *Journal of Personality and Social Psychology,* 77(2), 247–278.

[JELINEK2010] Jelinek, L., Stockbauer, C., Randjbar, S., et al. (2010). Characteristics and organization of the worst moment of trauma memories in posttraumatic stress disorder. *Behaviour Research and Therapy, 48*, 680–685.

[JETHAVA2022] Jethava, V., Kadish, J., Kakonge, L., and Wiseman-Hakes, C. (2022). Early attachment and the development of social communication: a neuropsychological approach. *Front Psychiatry 13*, 838950. *https://doi. org/10.3389/fpsyt.2022.838950*

[JOHNSON2005] Johnson, M. H. (2005). Subcortical face processing. *Nature Reviews Neuroscience, 6*, 766–774. doi: 10.1038/nrn1766.

[KAMILOGLU2021] Kamiloglu, R. G., and Sauter, D. A. (2021). Voice production and perception. In O. Braddick (Ed.), *Oxford Research Encyclopedia of Psychology [e-766].* Oxford England: Oxford University Press.

[KASHDAN2010] Kashdan, T. B., Ferssizidis, P., Collins, R. L., and Muraven, M. (2010). Emotion differentiation as resilience against excessive alcohol use: An ecological momentary assessment in underage social drinkers. *Psychological Science, 21(9)*, 1341–1347.

[KISSLER2006] Kissler, J., Assadollahi, R., and Herbert, C. (2006). Emotional and semantic networks in visual word processing: insights from ERP studies. *Progress in Brain Research, 156*, 147–183. doi: 10.1016/ S0079-6123(06)56008-X

[KOTZ2007] Kotz, S. A., and Paulmann, S. (2007). When emotional prosody and semantics dance cheek to cheek: ERP evidence. *Brain Research,* 1151, 107–118. doi: 10.1016/j.brainres.2007.03.015

[KREITLER2002] Kreitler, S. (2002). The psychosemantic approach to alexithymia. *Personality and Individual Differences, 33*, 393–407.

[LANE1987] Lane, R. D, and Schwartz, G. E., (1987). Levels of emotional awareness: a cognitive developmental theory and its application to psychopathology. *The American Journal of Psychiatry, (144)*, 133–143.

[LECLERE2014] Leclère C, Viaux S, Avril M, Achard C, Chetouani M, Missonnier S, et al. (2014) Why synchrony matters during mother-child interactions: a systematic review. *PLoS One* (9).

[LEDOUX1984] LeDoux, J. E., Sakaguchi, A., and Reis, D. J. (1984). Subcortical efferent projections of the medial geniculate nucleus mediate emotional responses conditioned to acoustic stimuli. *J. Neurosci.* 4, 683–698

[LEDOUX2000] LeDoux, J. E. (2000). Emotion circuits in the brain. *Annu. Rev. Neurosci.* 23, 155–184. doi: 10.1146/annurev.neuro.23.1.155

[LENNARZ2018] Lennarz, H. K., Lichtwarck-Aschoff, A., Timmerman, M. E., & Granic, I. (2018). Emotion differentiation and its relation with emotional well-being in adolescents. *Cognition and Emotion, 32(3)*, 651–657.

[LEWIS2007] Lewis, P. A., Critchley, H. D., Rotshtein, P., and Dolan, R. J. (2007). Neural correlates of processing valence and arousal in affective words. *Cereb. Cortex* 17, 742–748. doi: 10.1093/cercor/bhk024

[LIEBENTHAL2014] Liebenthal, E., Desai, R. H., Humphries, C., Sabri, M., and Desai, A. (2014). The functional organization of the left STS:a large scale meta-analysis of PET and fMRI studies of healthy adults. *Front. Neurosci.* 8:289. doi: 10.3389/fnins.2014.00289

[LIEBENTHAL2016] Liebenthal E., Silbersweig D.A., Stern E. (2016). The Language, Tone and Prosody of Emotions: Neural Substrates and Dynamics of Spoken-Word Emotion Perception, *Frontiers in Neuroscience, (10).*

[LINDQUIST2006] Lindquist, K. A., Barrett, L. F., Bliss-Moreau, E., & Russell, J. A. (2006). Language and the perception of emotion. *Emotion, 6(1)*, 125–138.

[LIU2000] Liu, C. H., Collin, C. A., Rainville, S. J., and Chaudhuri, A. (2000). The effects of spatial frequency overlap on face recognition. *J. Exp. Psychol. Hum. Percept. Perform.* 26, 956–979. doi: 10.1037/0096-1523.26.3.956

[LIVINGSTONE1988] Livingstone, M., and Hubel, D. (1988). Segregation of form, color, movement, and depth: anatomy, physiology, and perception. *Science* 240, 740–749. doi: 10.1126/science.3283936

[LOBNER2011] Löbner, S. (2011). Concept types and determination. Journal of Semantics, 28, 279-333.

[LUMINET2004] Luminet, O., Rimé, B., Bagby, R. M., et al. (2004). A multimodal investigation of emotional responding in alexithymia. Cognition and Emotion, 18, 741-766

[LURIA1966] Luria AR. (1966) *Human Brain and Psychological Processes.* trans. B. Haigh. New York, NY: Harper and Row

[MATTES2019] Mattes, J. (2019). Systematic review and meta-analysis of correlates of FFMQ mindfulness facets. *Frontiers in Psychology, 10,* Article 2684. *https://doi.org/10.3389/fpsyg.2019.02684*

[MATTHEWS2018] Matthews D, B H, Abbot-Smith K. (2018). Individual differences in children's pragmatic ability: a review of associations with formal language, social cognition, and executive functions. *Lang Learn Dev. (14)* 186–223.

[MCFAYDEN1996] McFadyen RG, Kitson WJ. (1996). Language comprehension and expression among adolescents who have experienced childhood physical abuse. *J Child Psychol Psychiat.* (37) 551–62.

[MEINS2002] Meins E, Fernyhough C, Wainwright R, Das Gupta M, Fradley E, Tuckey M. (2002). Maternal mind-mindedness and attachment security as predictors of theory of mind understanding. *Child Dev.* (2002) 73:1715–26.

[MERIGAN1993] Merigan, W. H., and Maunsell, J. H. (1993). How parallel are the primate visual pathways? *Annu. Rev. Neurosci.* 16, 369–402.

[MITCHELL2003] Mitchell, R. L., Elliott, R., Barry, M., Cruttenden, A., and Woodruff, P. W. (2003). The neural response to emotional prosody, as revealed by functional magnetic resonance imaging. *Neuropsychologia* 41, 1410–1421. doi: 10.1016/S0028-3932(03)00017-4

[MOLL2010] Moll H, Tomasello M. (2010) Infant cognition. *Curr Biol.* (20) R872–5.

[MOLL2021] Moll H, Pueschel E, Ni Q, Little A. (2021) Sharing experiences in infancy: from primary intersubjectivity to shared intentionality. *Front Psychol.* (12) 667-679.

[MORALES2000] Morales M, Mundy P, Delgado CE, Yale M, Messinger D, Neal R, et al. (2000) Responding to joint attention across the 6-through 24-month age period and early language acquisition. *J Appl Dev Psychol.* (21) 283–98.

[MORRIS1999] Morris, J. S., Scott, S. K., and Dolan, R. J. (1999). Saying it with feeling: neural responses to emotional vocalizations. *Neuropsychologia* 37, 1155–1163. doi: 10.1016/S0028-3932(99)00015-9

[MUNDY2006] Mundy PC, Acra C. (2006) Joint attention, social engagement, and the development of social competence. In: Marshall PJ, Fox NA. editors. *The Development of Social Engagement: Neurobiological Perspectives.* New York, NY: Oxford University Press; p. 81–117.

[MUNDY2017] Mundy P. (2017) A review of joint attention and social-cognitive brain systems in typical development and autism spectrum disorder. *Eur J Neurosci.* (1) 18. 10.1111/ejn.13720

[NAKIC2006] Nakic, M., Smith, B. W., Busis, S., Vythilingam, M., and Blair, R. J. (2006). The impact of affect and frequency on lexical decision: the role of the amygdala and inferior frontal cortex. *Neuroimage* 31, 1752–1761. doi: 10.1016/j.neuroimage.2006.02.022

[NEMIAH1970] Nemiah, J. C. and Sifneos, P. E. (1970). Psychosomatic illness: A problem in communication. *Psychotherapy and Psychosomatics, 18*, 154-160.

[NEMIAH1976] Nemiah J.C., Freyberger, H., and Sifneos, P.E. (1976). Alexithymia: A view of the psychosomatic process. In O.W. Hill (Ed.), *Modern Trends in Psychosomatic Medicine, Vol. 3*, pp. 430-439. London: Butterworths

[NEUHOFF19998] Neuhoff, J. G. (1998). Perceptual bias for rising tones. *Nature* 395, 123–124. doi: 10.1038/25862

[NOESSELT2002] Noesselt, T., Hillyard, S. A., Woldorff, M. G., Schoenfeld, A., Hagner, T., Jäncke, L., et al. (2002). Delayed striate cortical activation during spatial attention. *Neuron* 35, 575–587. doi: 10.1016/S0896-6273(02)00781-X

[NYGARD2008] Nygaard, L. C., and Queen, J. S. (2008). Communicating emotion: linking affective prosody and word meaning. *J. Exp. Psychol. Hum. Percept. Perform.* 34, 1017–1030. doi: 10.1037/0096-1523.34.4.1017

[OLSSON2004] Olsson, A., and Phelps, E. A. (2004). Learned fear of "unseen" faces after Pavlovian, observational, and instructed fear. *Psychol. Sci.* 15, 822–828. doi: 10.1111/j.0956-7976.2004.00762.x

[PAEZ1999] Páez, D., Velasco, C. and González, J. L. (1999). Expressive writing and the role of alexythimia as a dispositional deficit in self-disclosure and psychological health. Journal of Personality and Social Psychology, 77, 630

[PEGNA2005] Pegna, A. J., Khateb, A., Lazeyras, F., and Seghier, M. L. (2005). Discriminating emotional faces without primary visual cortices involves the right amygdala. *Nat. Neurosci.* 8, 24–25. doi: 10.1038/nn1364

[PELL2011] Pell, M. D., and Kotz, S. A. (2011). On the time course of vocal emotion recognition. *PLoS ONE* 6:e27256. doi: 10.1371/journal.pone.0027256

[PELL2015] Pell, M. D., Rothermich, K., Liu, P., Paulmann, S., Sethi, S., and Rigoulot, S. (2015). Preferential decoding of emotion from human non-linguistic vocalizations versus speech prosody. *Biol. Psychol.* 111, 14–25. doi: 10.1016/j.biopsycho.2015.08.008

[PEZAWAS2005] Pezawas, L., Meyer-Lindenberg, A., Drabant, E. M., Verchinski, B. A., Munoz, K. E., Kolachana, B. S., et al. (2005). 5-HTTLPR polymorphism impacts human cingulate-amygdala interactions: a genetic susceptibility mechanism for depression. *Nat. Neurosci.* 8, 828–834. doi: 10.1038/nn1463

[PHELPS2001] Phelps, E. A., O'Connor, K. J., Gatenby, J. C., Gore, J. C., Grillon, C., and Davis, M. (2001). Activation of the left amygdala to a cognitive representation of fear. *Nat. Neurosci.* 4, 437–441. doi: 10.1038/86110

[PHELPS2005] Phelps, E. A., and LeDoux, J. E. (2005). Contributions of the amygdala to emotion processing: from animal models to human behavior. *Neuron* 48, 175–187. doi: 10.1016/j.neuron.2005.09.025

[PHILLIPS1998] Phillips, M. L., Young, A. W., Scott, S. K., Calder, A. J., Andrew, C., Giampietro, V., et al. (1998). Neural responses to facial and vocal expressions of fear and disgust. *Proc. Biol. Sci.* 265, 1809–1817. doi: 10.1098/rspb.1998.0506

[POEPPEL2008] Poeppel, D., Idsardi, W. J., and van Wassenhove, V. (2008). Speech perception at the interface of neurobiology and linguistics. *Philos. Trans. R. Soc. Lond. B Biol. Sci.* 363, 1071–1086. doi: 10.1098/rstb.2007.2160

[POND2012] Pond, R. S., Jr., Kashdan, T. B., DeWall, C. N., Savostyanova, A., Lambert, N. M., & Fincham, F. D. (2012). Emotion differentiation moderates aggressive tendencies in angry people: A daily diary analysis. *Emotion, 12(2)*, 326–337.

[POSNER2009] Posner, J., Russell, J. A., Gerber, A., Gorman, D., Colibazzi, T., Yu, S., et al. (2009). The neurophysiological bases of emotion: an fMRI study of the affective circumplex using emotion-denoting words. *Hum. Brain Mapp.* 30, 883–895. doi: 10.1002/hbm.20553

[POURTOIS2004] Pourtois, G., Grandjean, D., Sander, D., and Vuilleumier, P. (2004). Electrophysiological correlates of rapid spatial orienting towards fearful faces. *Cereb. Cortex* 14, 619–633. doi: 10.1093/cercor/bhh023

[PROTOPOPESCU2005] Protopopescu, X., Pan, H., Tuescher, O., Cloitre, M., Goldstein, M., Engelien, W., et al. (2005). Differential time courses and specificity of amygdala activity in posttraumatic stress disorder subjects and normal control subjects. *Biol. Psychiatry* 57, 464–473. doi: 10.1016/j.biopsych.2004.12.026

[REDDY2015] Reddy, V. (2015) Joining intentions in infancy. *The Journal of Consciousness, (22)*, 24–44.

[RICE2022] Rice, A., Lavender, J. M., Shank, L. M., Higgins Neyland, M. K., Markos, B., Repke, H., Haynes, H., Gallagher-Teske, J., Schvey, N. A., Sbrocco, T., Wilfley, D. E., Ford, B., Ford, C. B., Jorgensen, S., Yanovski, J. A., Haigney, M., Klein, D. A., Quinlan, J., and Tanofsky-Kraff, M. (2022). Associations among alexithymia, disordered eating, and depressive symptoms in treatment-seeking adolescent military dependents at risk for adult binge-eating disorder and obesity. *Eating and weight disorders: EWD, 27*(8), 3083–3093. *https://doi.org/10.1007/s40519-022-01429-z*

[RIEFFE2007] Rieffe, C., Terwogt, M. M., Petrides, K. V., Cowan, R., Miers, A. C., and Tolland, A. (2007). Psychometric properties of the Emotion Awareness Questionnaire for children. *Personality and Individual Differences, 43(1)*, 95–105.

[ROEDEMA1999] Roedema, T. M. and Simons, R. F. (1999). Emotion-processing deficit in alexithymia. *Psychophysiology, 36*, 379–387.

[ROSENKRANZ2003] Rosenkranz, J. A., Moore, H., and Grace, A. A. (2003). The prefrontal cortex regulates lateral amygdala neuronal plasticity and responses to previously conditioned stimuli. *The Journal of Neuroscience*, 23, 11054–11064.

[RUSSELL1986] Russell, J. A., and Bullock, M. (1986). On the dimensions, preschoolers use to interpret facial expressions of emotion. *Developmental Psychology, 22(1)*, 97–102.

[SAARNI1997] Saarni, C. (1997). Coping with aversive feelings. *Motivation and Emotion, 21* (1), 45–63. doi:10.1023/A:1024474314409

[SAMUR2018] Samur, D. Language Processing in Alexithymia Chapter · September 2018 doi: 10.1017/9781108241595.008

[SANDER2001] Sander, K., and Scheich, H. (2001). Auditory perception of laughing and crying activates human amygdala regardless of attentional state. *Brain Research Cognitive Brain Research*, 12, 81–198. doi: 10.1016/S0926-6410(01)00045-3

[SANDER2003] Sander, K., Brechmann, A., and Scheich, H. (2003b). Audition of laughing and crying leads to right amygdala activation in a low-noise fMRI setting. *Brain Research. Brain Research Protocols. 11*, 81–91.

[SANDER2003A] Sander, D., Grafman, J., and Zalla, T. (2003a). The human amygdala: an evolved system for relevance detection. *Reviews in the Neurosciences, 14,* 303–316.

[SANDER2005] Sander, D., Grandjean, D., Pourtois, G., Schwartz, S., Seghier, M. L., Scherer, K. R., et al. (2005). Emotion and attention interactions in social cognition: brain regions involved in processing anger prosody. *Neuroimage, 28,* 848–858. doi: 10.1016/j.neuroimage.2005.06.023

[SCHACHT2009] Schacht, A., and Sommer, W. (2009). Time course and task dependence of emotion effects in word processing. *Cognitive, Affective, & Behavioral Neuroscience, 9,* 28–43. doi: 10.3758/CABN.9.1.28

[SCHOLMERICH1997] Schölmerich, A., Lamb, M., Leyendecker, B., and Fracasso M.P. (1997). Mother-infant teaching interactions and attachment security in Euro-American and Central-American immigrant families. *Infant Behavior and Development. (20),* 165–174. 10.1016/s0163-6383(97)90019-9

[SCHORE2008] Schore, A. (2008). Effects of a secure attachment relationship on right brain development, affect regulation and infant mental health, Department of Psychiatry and Biobehavioral Sciences University of California at Los Angeles School of Medicine.

[SCOTT1997] Scott, S. K., Young, A. W., Calder, A. J., Hellawell, D. J., Aggleton, J. P., and Johnson, M. (1997). Impaired auditory recognition of fear and anger following bilateral amygdala lesions. *Nature, 385,* 254–257. doi: 10.1038/385254a0

[SCOTT2009] Scott, G. G., O'Donnell, P. J., Leuthold, H., and Sereno, S. C. (2009). Early emotion word processing: evidence from event-related potentials. *Biological Psychology, 80,* 95–104. doi: 10.1016/j.biopsycho.2008.03.010

[SERGERIE2008] Sergerie, K., Chochol, C., and Armony, J. L. (2008). The role of the amygdala in emotional processing: a quantitative meta-analysis of functional neuroimaging studies. *Neuroscience & Biobehavioral Reviews, 32,* 811–830. doi: 10.1016/j.neubiorev.2007.12.002

[SHABLACK2019] Shablack, H., Becker, M., and Lindquist, K. A. (2019). How do children learn novel emotion? words? A study of emotion concept acquisition in preschoolers. *Journal of Experimental Psychology: General, 149(8),* 1537–1553.

[SIEGEL2012] Siegel, D. J., and Bryson, P. H. D. T. P. (2012). *The Whole-Brain Child.* New York: Random House.

[TAUMOEPEAU2006] Taumoepeau, M., and Ruffman, T. (2006). Mother and infant talk about mental states relates to desire language and emotion understanding. *Child Development,* (77), 465–81. 10.1111/j.1467-8624.2006.00882.x

[TAYLOR1991] Taylor, G. J., Bagby, R. M., and Parker, J. D. A (1991). The alexithymia construct: A potential paradigm for psychosomatic medicine. *Psychosomatics,* (32), 2. 153-164,

[TAYLOR2000] Taylor, G. J. (2000). Recent developments in alexithymia theory and research. *Canadian Journal of Psychiatry,* (45), 134–142. *https://doi.org/10.1177/070674370004500203*

[THOMAS2007] Thomas, S. J., Johnstone, S. J., and Gonsalvez, C. J. (2007). Event-related potentials during an emotional Stroop task. *International Journal of Psychophysiology,* 63, 221–231. doi: 10.1016/j.ijpsycho.2006.10.002

[TOMAS2019] Tomas, E., and Vissers C. (2019). Behind the scenes of developmental language disorder: time to call neuropsychology back on stage. *Frontiers in Human Neuroscience,* (12) 517. 10.3389/fnhum.2018.00517.

[TOMASELLO2005] Tomasello M. Understanding and sharing intentions. *Behaviour of Brain Science,* 28, 675–91. 10.1017/S0140525X05000129

[TOMASELLO2019] Tomasello, M. (2019). *Becoming Human: A Theory of Ontogeny.* Cambridge, MA: Belknap Press.

[TREVARTHEN2001] Trevarthen, C., and Aitken, K.J. (2001) Infant intersubjectivity: Research, theory, and clinical applications. *Journal of Child Psychology and Psychiatry,* (42), 3–48. 10.1111/1469-7610.00701

[TSUCHIYA2009] Tsuchiya, N., Moradi, F., Felsen, C., Yamazaki, M., and Adolphs, R. (2009). Intact rapid detection of fearful faces in the absence of the amygdala. *Nature Neuroscience,* 12, 1224–1225. doi: 10.1038/nn.2380

[TUGADE2004] Tugade, M. M., Fredrickson, B. L., and Barrett, L. F. (2004). Psychological resilience and positive emotional granularity: Examining the benefits of positive emotions on coping and health. *Journal of Personalized,* 72(6), 1161–1190.

[TULL2005] Tull, M. T., Medaglia, E., and Roemer, L. (2005). An investigation of the construct validity of the 20-Item Toronto Alexithymia Scale through the use of a verbalization task. *Journal of Psychosomatic Research,* 59, 77–84.

[VALLOTTON2010] Vallotton, C. D., and Ayoub, C. C. (2010). Symbols build communication and thought: the role of gestures and words in the development of engagement skills and social-emotional concepts during toddlerhood. *Soc Development,* 19, 601–626. 10.1111/j.1467-9507.2009.00549.x

[VANHEULE2011] Vanheule, S., Meganck, R., and Desmet, M. (2011). Alexithymia, social detachment and cognitive processing. *Psychiatry Research, 190,* 49–51.

[VISSERS2016] Vissers, C., and Koolen, S. (2016). Theory of mind deficits and social emotional functioning in preschoolers with specific language impairment. *Frontiers in Psychology,* 7, 1734. 10.3389/fpsyg.2016.01734

[VISSERS2020] Vissers, C. T. W., Tomas, E., and Law, J. (2020). The emergence of inner speech and its measurement in atypically developing children. *Frontiers in Psychology, (11),* 279. 10.3389/fpsyg.2020.00279

[VUILLEUMIER2003] Vuilleumier, P., Armony, J. L., Driver, J., and Dolan, R. J. (2003). Distinct spatial frequency sensitivities for processing faces and emotional expressions. *Nature Neuroscience,* 6, 624–631. doi: 10.1038/nn1057

[VUILLEUMIER2005] Vuilleumier, P., Schwartz, S., Duhoux, S., Dolan, R. J., and Driver, J. (2005). Selective attention modulates neural substrates of repetition priming and "implicit" visual memory: suppressions and enhancements revealed by FMRI. *Journal of Cognitive Neuroscience,* 17, 1245–1260. doi: 10.1162/0898929055002409

[VYGOTSKY1934] Vygotsky, L. S. (1934). *Thought and Language.* Moscow-Leningrad: Sotsekgiz.

[VYGOTSKY2012] Vygotsky, L. S. (2012). *Thought and Language: Revised and Expanded Edition.* Cambridge, MA: MIT Press.

[WAGNER2008] Wagner, H., and Lee, V. (2008). Alexithymia and individual differences in emotional expression. *Journal of Research in Personality,* 42, 83–95.

[WARRINER2013] Warriner, A. B., Kuperman, V., and Brysbaert, M. (2013). Norms of valence, arousal, and dominance for 13,915 English lemmas. *Behavior Research Methods,* 45, 1191–1207. doi: 10.3758/s13428-012-0314-x

[WEST2011] West, G. L., Anderson, A. A., Ferber, S., and Pratt, J. (2011). Electrophysiological evidence for biased competition in V1 for fear expressions. *Journal of Cognitive Neuroscience, 23,* 3410–3418. doi: 10.1162/jocn.2011.21605

[WESTBY2014] Westby, C., and Robinson, L. (2014). A developmental perspective for promoting theory of mind. *Top Language Learning Discord Servers (34),* 362–382.

[WHALEN2004] Whalen, P. J., Kagan, J., Cook, R. G., Davis, F. C., Kim, H., Polis, S., et al. (2004). Human amygdala responsivity to masked fearful eye whites. *Science,* 306, 2061. doi: 10.1126/science.1103617

[WIDEN2003] Widen, S. C., and Russell, J. A. (2003). A closer look at preschoolers' freely produced labels for facial expressions. *Developmental Psychology, 39(1),* 114–128.

[WIDEN2008] Widen, S. C., and Russell, J. A. (2008). Children acquire emotion categories gradually. *Cognitive Development, 23(2),* 291–312.

[WIDEN2013] Widen, S. C. (2013). Children's interpretation of facial expressions: The long path from valencebased to specific discrete categories. *Emotion Review, 5(1),* 72–77.

[WINSTON2003] Winston, J. S., O'Doherty, J., and Dolan, R. J. (2003). Common and distinct neural responses during direct and incidental processing of multiple facial emotions. *Neuroimage* 20, 84–97. Doi: 10.1016/S1053-8119(03)00303-3

[WOTSCHACK2013] Wotschack, C., and Klann-Delius, G. (2013). Alexithymia and the conceptualization of emotions: A study of language use and semantic knowledge. Journal of Research in Personality, 47, 514-523.

[WRIGHT2001] Wright, C. I., Fischer, H., Whalen, P. J., McInerney, S. C., Shin, L. M., and Rauch, S. L. (2001). Differential prefrontal cortex and amygdala habituation to repeatedly presented emotional stimuli. *Neuroreport* 12, 379–383. doi: 10.1097/00001756-200102120-00039

[WISEMAN2020]. Wiseman-Hakes, C., Kakonge, L., Doherty, M., and Beauchamp, M. A. (2020). Conceptual framework of social communication: clinical applications to pediatric traumatic brain injury. *Seminars in Speech and Language, 41,* 143–160.

[WRIGHT2001] Wright, C. I., Fischer, H., Whalen, P. J., McInerney, S. C., Shin, L. M., and Rauch, S. L. (2001). Differential prefrontal cortex and amygdala habituation to repeatedly presented emotional stimuli. *Neuroreport, 12,* 379–383. doi: 10.1097/00001756-200102120-00039

[WOODRUFF1978] Woodruff, G., and Premack, D. (1978). Does the chimpanzee have a theory of mind. *Behavioral and Brain Sciences.*1(4), 515–526.

[YANIV2021] Yaniv, A. U., Salomon, R., Waidergoren, S., Shimon-Raz, O., Djalovski, A., and Feldman, R. (2021). Synchronous caregiving from birth to adulthood tunes humans' social brain. *Proceedings of the National Academy of Sciences of the United States of America, 118(14),* Article e2012900118. *https://doi.org/10.1073/pnas.2012900118.*

[YEHUDA2005] Yehuda, N. A. (2005). The language of dissociation. *Journal of Trauma* & *Dissociation, 6(1),* 9–29.

[ZATORRE2001] Zatorre, R. J., and Belin, P. (2001). Spectral and temporal processing in human auditory cortex. *Cerebral Cortex,* 11, 946–953.

[ZIMMERMAN2006] Zimmermann, G. (2006). Delinquency in male adolescents: the role of alexithymia and family structure. *Journal of Adolescence,* 29, 321–332. doi: 10.1016/j.adolescence.2005.08.001

8

THE ROLE OF MATURITY, EXECUTIVE FUNCTIONING, AND SOCIAL UNDERSTANDING IN COMMUNICATION

Do you remember how the people around you talked about their problems or emotions when you were little? What types of words and phrases did they use to describe the people and situations they encountered? Do you notice any similarities between what you hear around you and your own inner dialogue? How do you feel about your ability to accurately perceive and understand others' internal states and intentions? In this chapter, we will dive into the human ability to understand the experiences and perspectives of other humans as a key to communication. This process reflects a developmental journey from immaturity to maturity and complexity. That journey begins, as we saw from previous chapters, with an inability to self-regulate and a dependence on other humans to attune to our biological needs of nutrition, shelter, and physical safety, as well as our socio physiological needs for attunement, connection, and freedom to explore and become autonomous beings. In the earliest phases of the maturation process, nonverbal transmissions and exchanges between infant and caregiver are critical. Those nonverbal exchanges lay a foundation for human communication and are transmitted via frequencies emitted from our facial muscles, vocal systems, and internal organs that affect many other subtle nonverbal transmissions. As humans mature, new abilities develop that help us bridge the nonverbal realm of visceral and sensory fluctuations with the verbal, symbolic dimension of words and gestures. The inability to verbally nuance our emotional states can lead to dysregulation, ineffective communication with others, and maladaptive strategies to attempt to regulate our state. In this chapter, we will continue to explore how language plays a central role in our ability not only to self-regulate but to understand other human beings. This complex level of understanding is key to effective communication. Without understanding others' intentions, patterns, and internal states, our communicative behaviors lack feedback responsiveness and context sensitivity. The ability to mentalize and internalize how other people think and feel provides data for our own internal system to respond to challenges and opportunities present in our social interactions. We will look at various developmental and social-communication researchers' perspectives on how social understanding intertwines with self-regulation, executive function, and language.

THE COMPLEXITY OF SOCIAL UNDERSTANDING

The sophistication, granularity, and complexity of communication and the ability to understand each other's intentions, behaviors, and internal states can attain levels in humans that are unmatched in any other species in the animal kingdom [TOMASELLO2005; FERNYHOUGH2008]. We saw in the previous chapter from studies on chimpanzees and young children that human language abilities play a key role in advancing human children's ability to solve problems and understand conspecific behavior. These abilities draw on a level of consciousness that acknowledges other humans as intentional agents who have their own perspectives and agendas but who can join their attention on common objects—features of what is called social understanding (SU). Various theories have emerged to explain how SU develops and how it manifests. The field of simulation theory proposes that SU requires an ability to use the imagination to project oneself into the perspective of another and create a simulation of what they are thinking [GORDON1992; HARRIS1989]. Within this framework, a child's imaginative capacities would set limits on their ability to simulate sociocognitive processes [FERNYHOUGH2008]. Another theory proposes that SU depends on the ability to represent and process narratives [LEWIS1994]. A third theory relates to intention-sharing. Tomasello and colleagues highlight that humans have a species-specific motivation to share intentional states with others, and that this process builds sophisticated sociocognitive networks needed to understand others' behaviors and thought processes [TOMASELLO2005; FERNYHOUGH2008].

Social Understanding and Language

As stated in Chapter 7, language plays a vital role in developing SU. Extensive empirical evidence shows how children's conceptual understanding of other minds increases as their linguistic skills become more complex and sophisticated [ASTINGTON2005]. As researchers continue to see a connection between language and SU, there is a parallel increase in exploring how language and cognition in general are interrelated [CLARK2006]. The connection between language and cognition is an evolution from previous models that considered them as separate categories. The connections between language and children's ability to understand other minds, has also led to a reemergence of interest in the work of Vygotsky, Mead, and Luria—important figures in the history of developmental psychology [FERNYHOUGH2008].

Strong research evidence proposes that a child's ability to understand others is determined by their ability to conceive of and activate social-cognitive neural resources that they already have and that these resources develop in parallel with the social influences they have around them [FERNYHOUGH2008]. This makes SU similar in sensitivity to social and environmental experiences and surroundings as the self-regulating and executive functioning processes mentioned in previous chapters. What SU and executive functioning (EF) research further reveals is that this sensitivity to social experiences is also specifically tied to linguistic input [FERNYHOUGH2008]. Multiple factors play a role in this social-context input and how SU develops in individuals.

Some of these factors include:

- Mental-state talk: caregivers' use of language to describe mental states (versus behavior) [DOAN2010] and causality of feelings [DUNN1991] is associated with children's ability to understand the emotional state of others.

- Family size and interaction: theory of mind abilities in children is influenced by the number of interactions with adult kin as well as the number of older siblings a child interacts with, suggesting that having knowledgeable social influences plays a role in developing an understanding of others' minds [LEWIS1996].

- Attachment security: superior mentalizing abilities have been found in children who were assessed as having a secure attachment to their caregivers [MEINS1998]. These secure-related differences are potentially related to caregivers' use of sensitive tutoring strategies and a higher likelihood of describing their children in terms of mental characteristics (as opposed to behavior or appearance) [MEINS1998].

- Mind-mindedness: children's performance on Theory of Mind tasks has shown to be positively correlated with mother's use of mental-state language that appropriately reflects an infant's state (compared with language that does not appropriately reflect it) [MEINS2002].

Language as a Cognitive Niche and Psychological Tool

One perspective of how language and cognition influence each other is to look at language as a cognitive niche [CLARK2006]. As defined by Clark, a cognitive niche is a type of thought-enabling, cognition-enhancing, animal-built structure that moves a problem into an external physical space in ways that help thinking and reasoning [CLARK2006]. Language materializes thought into a physical presence of sounds in the air or words on a page, which can then become objects that we can perceive, manipulate, and think *about* (rather than just think), thus reconfiguring our cognitive workspace and attention to accommodate these externalized objects [CLARK2006; CLARK1998]. These physical structures can then be combined and influenced by cultural and social factors, making entirely new forms of thought and problem-solving possible [CLARK2006]. Language is like a layer of material structure that we encounter in the world of senses. These structures not only play a communicative role but can also serve as self-stimulating processes that help humans enhance cognition, augment learning, and scaffold their own behavior by helping distribute attention and mediate our recall of information [CLARK2006; HERMER1999].

Other perspectives on language and thought stem from developmental psychologists influenced by the works of Mead [MEAD1934], Luria [LURIA1965], and Vygotsky [1978; 1987]. Vygotsky proposed that words are a type of "psychological tool" that creates an entirely new class of higher mental functions by reshaping brain processes [FERNYHOUGH2008; VYGOTSKY1978; 1987]. In his work on examining the connections between social interaction, SU, and EF, Charles Fernyhough highlights the importance of Vygotsky's inter-functional approach to understanding that language, biology, and social environment are all bidirectionally influencing each other and affect our communication and self-regulation abilities [FERNYHOUGH2008]. Vygotsky proposed that children gain self-regulating control over their behavior when words that were once shared with and heard by others become reformulated into an internal activity. Specifically, words that children have heard others use to regulate their own behavior, or to regulate the behavior of others, become internalized into a process of regulating the self [FERNYHOUGH2008].

This model suggests that linguistic abilities that are initially shared with others are reformulated into a different type of mental process. In this process, prelinguistic abilities associated with EF, such as monitoring, planning, and inhibitory control, begin to interrelate with language abilities [FERNYHOUGH2008]. In this line of reasoning, natural and prelinguistic developmental processes become interwoven with cultural, language-based, and social experiences, all of which influence self-regulating abilities through a progressive internalization of verbal interactions with others [FERNYHOUGH2008; WINSLER2009]. Empirical research supports the idea that elementary forms of executive function such as monitoring, planning, and inhibition exist in children before the development of language, and that through verbal social interaction, these abilities become incorporated into new functional self-regulatory systems [WINSLER2003; DIAMOND1991; FERNYHOUGH2008]. Research by Wertsch and colleagues [WERTSCH1985] offers evidence that there is a progressive transfer from adult to child of responsibilities for strategizing as children internalize verbal dialogue they have shared previously with adults in problem-solving contexts as a mechanism for solving their own problems.

Private and Inner Speech

An important part of Vygotsky's theories that support this internalization of verbal self-regulation is related to children's private and inner speech. Private speech is speech that can be heard by others but is not addressed to another person [WINSLER2004]. Inner speech is not audible to others—it is fully internal verbal thought [WINSLER2009]. Because it is audible, children's private speech offers an avenue of research that can be empirically studied and integrated with children's various social experiences and influences [FERNYHOUGH2008]. According to Vygotsky, from the moment of birth, infants are bathed in social exchanges that include words, and as the infant's own linguistic abilities develop, these words are turned back on the self and mediate their own thought processes and behaviors [FERNYHOUGH2008]. In the early years of life, this private speech is mainly audible and overt but over time becomes completely covert, internal, and inaudible, transforming into inner speech [FERNYHOUGH2008]. Over the years, an emergence of empirical studies has supported this theory [BERK1992; WINSLER2004]. Some of these studies reveal a developmental trajectory of language activity that validates the progression of private speech in early preschool years into inner speech in later childhood [KOHLBERG1968; WINSLER2003].

Another element of Vygotsky's framework that has been supported by research is the connection between private speech and a child's ability to perform a task. This is particularly reflected in studies showing that private speech is at its highest when a task appropriately matches a child's competency level [KOHLBERG2003; FRAUENGLASS1985]. Other research has shown that social influences on private speech development in children affect cognitive facilitation and that private speech aids in selective attention abilities that lead preschoolers to be more successful on task than children who do not engage in private speech [WINSLER1997]. In connection with language and higher-order mental processes, children's executive function performance has also been associated with verbal abilities [CARLSON2004; HUGHES2005; PERNER2002]. In attentional control tasks, preschool children who verbally label the task as they perform it had better performance outcomes than non-labeling children [MULLER2004].

The connections between executive function, SU, and internalized speech suggest that as children participate in activities with more expert partners, they develop an internal dialogue that will help them master those activities [WERTSCH1985; FERNYHOUGH2008]. When adequate language needed for regulatory control is developed, inner speech can also serve as a tool for self-regulation [FERNYHOUGH1996]. The internal dialogues that develop in children depend on how the adults around them talk about problem-solving, processes, feelings, and experiences. As described in Chapter 9, some psychotherapeutic and psychoeducational approaches to improving mental health and quality of life have a basis in this internal speech and how we can take steps to update it and use it more effectively for personal growth, as well as improving relationships. Communication is a form of relaying our internal experiences outward. The more we can verbalize these experiences, the more accurately we are able to convey information to improve the effectiveness of our communication efforts. In alignment with this, several studies suggest that language ability is strongly correlated with SU [CUTTING1999; DEVILLIERS2000; JENKINS1996]. SU also appears to have some similarities with EF in that it is sensitive to environmental inputs and social experiences [FERNYHOUGH2010].

Exploring communication through the lens of functional integration of executive function, semiotics, self-regulation, and SU opens up an avenue for therapies and prevention studies that focus on developing adequate inner speech through social interactions. What we see from this integration of research involving language, executive function, and SU (or theory of mind) is that semiotics—the use of signs and symbols such as words—plays a role in mediating our ability to achieve internal state regulation as well as our ability to express, receive and process verbal information from others to integrate into our own neural and behavioral resources. Language enhances our access to higher mental functions and increases our repertoire of regulating strategies. Our social experiences influence the amount, quality, and variety of words we use to describe our internal and external worlds. The larger the variety and granularity of these descriptors, the wider range of explanations and interpretations we can give to what is happening. These higher-order elements of verbal range and repertoire are also tied to cognitive and explanatory flexibility.

COGNITIVE FLEXIBILITY AND COMMUNICATION

Another key concept tied to executive function is cognitive flexibility. Cognitive flexibility underlies the ability to direct attention in new ways to constantly changing, emergent stimuli. It involves ascertaining that a certain strategy is not suited to a current situation, inhibiting previous responses, and reconfiguring new behavioral strategies [DAJANI2015]. Cognitive flexibility relates to all forms of behavior, which includes communication. Without cognitive flexibility and its related EF abilities, communication would become ineffective as it would lack responsiveness to dynamically changing information. Cognitive flexibility is also associated with favorable outcomes in various domains of life, such as better reading abilities in childhood [DEABREU2014], increased resilience to negative life events [GENET2011], higher creative abilities [CHEN2014], and improved quality of life in older populations [DAVIS2010].

Research suggests that cognitive flexibility is enhanced through language. Some of these studies look at how humans conjoin geometric and nongeometric information to improve visuospatial abilities, compared with animals that only rely on the shape of an environment to reorient themselves [HERMER1999]. Humans' unique verbal abilities play a key role in cognitive flexibility by integrating diverse sources of information into one unitary unit that can be expressed and internalized [HERMER1999].

COGNITIVE PROCESSES AND DISTORTIONS

As we have explored in this chapter thus far, language and cognition play important roles in adaptive psychological functioning and social behavior, which includes communication. We have also focused on inner and private speech. In this section, we will look at some frameworks of language that tie together cognitive and linguistic processes and that relate to how humans associate meaning with stimuli and experiences. These processes also highlight the complexity and unique human level of sophistication found in semiotics. Some of these theories can also help elucidate cognitive rigidity found in some forms of psychopathology. To adequately cover all of these theories would require an entire book of its own; we will therefore outline a few that might help to deepen and expand our understanding of what has been covered thus far. Some of these include Relational Frame Theory, generic versus individuated language and self-disclosure.

Relational Frame Theory

To begin this exploration, we will look at some basic principles stemming from a theory of language called Relational Frame Theory (RFT), developed by Steven C. Hayes and later expanded on by various researchers such as Dermon Barnes-Holmes. RFT proposes that human language and cognition are founded in the human ability to create *relational links* between things [BLACKLEDGE2003]. Although this theory is complex and has been debated widely in research communities, it is a useful framework for exploring possibilities in how humans associate words with internal and external experiences. RFT highlights the human ability to create relational links between stimuli as a foundation of human language and cognition. [BLACKLEDGE2003]. We can deepen our understanding of communication when we look at how humans learn to associate certain words with meaning and how words can influence our worldview, perceptions, emotions, and behaviors.

Relational Frame Theory and the Lang Fear Network

RFT also has parallels to another important theory regarding human behavior: the Lang Fear Network. In the Lang Fear Network model, various components to stimuli form a schema in long-term memory [BLACKLEDGE2003]. These components include stimulus propositions, meaning propositions, and response propositions [BLACKLEDGE2003]. Stimulus propositions are the initial stimuli we encounter with our external and internal senses. Meaning propositions are activations of networks that imply that a stimulus means or represents something. Response propositions are the aspect of these neuro-behavioral schemas that include physiological responses and overt behaviors.

Only one of these components needs to be encountered in order for the entire schema to be activated [BLACKLEDGE2003]. These components can be learned through direct experience, instruction, or through modeling. An example of this can be demonstrated with a walk in a wooded area and the observation of a quick movement. In this scenario, the stimulus propositions offer the initial input (the wooded area, the movement). The implications of those stimuli are then influenced by the meaning propositions, such that seeing movement in a wooded area implies danger [BLACKLEDGE2003]. The response proposition would include accelerated heart rate, feeling afraid, and running away [BLACKLEDGE2003]. These components may have been learned through the direct experience of being hurt by something moving in a wooded area, or through instruction such as education about wild animals in the area, or modeling, such as seeing someone previously run away from the source of quick movement in a wooded area [BLACKLEDGE2003].

Lang's fear network is helpful in understanding RFT [BLACKLEDGE2003]. In the following example, we will continue to use the wooded area and snake scenario to illustrate how various connections are made between stimuli and response. While this example may seem unrelated to communication, its relevance is tied to the associations that may be made that could affect our reaction to a situation. What we will see in the following example is that we respond to stimuli for reasons that may not seem obvious or conscious but are rather comprised of associations and relational networks. The look on someone's face, a smell, a certain word, gesture, voice frequency—all of these are components of an overall schema of networks that associate with each other and can trigger a response such as a fight or flight, even without a stimulus that is in and of itself threatening. Understanding how these relational associations are made can help us understand our verbal and nonverbal responses during social interactions. In our example scenario, we will illustrate examples of thoughts, emotions, physiological sensations, and overt behavior as well as the implicit and explicit links between them [BLACKLEDGE2003]. We will use the wooded area and sudden movement to illustrate concepts from both RFT and the Lang Fear Network model.

Patterns of relational associations in RFT include coordination, opposition, distinction, comparison, hierarchy, and perspective-taking [HAYES2001]. Within the Lang Fear Network model, we see examples of three of these relationships: causal, coordination, and hierarchical. In our wooded area scenario, the feeling and sensations tied to being afraid can be considered as a cause for running away—highlighting a causal relationship. Seeing a snake and considering it dangerous would be a relationship of coordination or equivalence in the sense that "snake" is considered to be roughly equivalent to "danger." A hierarchical relationship exists between the stimuli of "snake" and "wooded area." In this case, the snake is part of something larger than it with unpredictable pathways for movement [BLACKLEDGE2003]. The hierarchical association in the wooded area is different than a hierarchical association that would be triggered by a snake inside an enclosed glass case at a zoo and would therefore activate a different type of schema.

One of the key principles of RFT is the importance of relationships between stimuli. For example, being in a wooded area might lead to a fear response depending on the associations that have been learned (directly or indirectly) about wooded areas and potential dangers. Notice how, when it comes to young children, they may need to receive instructions to pay attention and be alert to their surroundings because those fear networks have not yet been established. Because they have a shorter amount of time receiving inputs from their environment, their relational networks have fewer associations between stimuli.

While some responses and associations are learned, many linkages between stimuli emerge through experience and are therefore "derived." As a child has more and more experiences with one stimulus being related to another, they begin to derive a relationship between them. This is one of the foundations of RFT, called "derived relational responding." The term "derived" relates to a bidirectional linking between stimuli that emerge and are not taught [ZETTLE2016] If a learner is taught that stimulus A is the same as stimulus B, the bidirectional relation derived from this will be "B same as A." When children who are offered enough learning history and examples learn to orient toward their mother when they hear the word "mom," they may begin saying "mom" whenever their mother is present. This relation is bidirectional: learning to turn toward the mother when they hear the word "mom" is a word-person relation of coordination, whereas seeing the mother and then saying "mom" is a derived person-word coordination relation [ZETTLE2016]. Derived relational responding is considered a fundamental pillar to acquiring complex verbal repertoires as well as novel verbal responses and repertoires [ZETTLE2016]. Another example would be a child learning that the word chair applies to the object they are sitting in and then later learning that chair, seat, and stool are all similar. If they then use the word "seat" to describe a chair they are sitting in, this verbal response was not previously reinforced and is therefore derived [ZETTLE2016].

This is important for us to think about as we explore the realm of communication. If a goal is to improve our effectiveness with communication, understanding that we may be responding to associations we have with a stimulus may help us become more aware of how we can change or improve our response. Through our experiences, we develop networks associated with a certain tone of voice (stimulus proposition) or a person's position in our social hierarchy, such as a parent as an authority figure (their position of authority has an implied meaning for us, making it a meaning proposition), as well as response propositions associated with those network components. When we interact with someone who is not a parent but who is an authority figure, they may activate one of those network components and the associated responses. Another person may activate one of those schemas based on a stimulus such as tone of voice, posture, or smell. All of these linkages and associations we make during our interactions may therefore be based on earlier experiences and less attuned to the live, emergent information that is available to us now. What is important to note is that when communication is happening between people, this communication is often based on evaluations that are activated by these interplaying networks. These evaluations may be irrational or cause behavioral responses that lead to disruptions, distress, or conflict within communicative interactions with others [MALKINSON2013].

Cognitive Therapies

These types of triggered responses that distort our present-moment perception relate to theories of biased information processing and cognitive distortions that form the basis of many psychotherapies today, particularly cognitive behavioral therapies and adapted versions of it. Two of the most influential psychologists who have influenced these cognitive therapies are Aaron Beck and Albert Ellis. Beck's cognitive theories were based on his proposal that treatments for depression were based too heavily on past events, rather than patients' current beliefs about the event [BECK2011]. The ABC model proposed by Ellis parallels RFT and Lang's Fear Network. In this model, behavioral responses or consequences (C) are not directly activated by an event (A), but rather our beliefs and how we cognitively process and evaluate the event (B) [OLTEAN2017].

Generic Versus Nongeneric Language

In addition to these relational associations between various components of stimuli, meaning, and responses, certain types of language and words can affect our perception, attitudes, and behaviors. Therapies, such as cognitive behavioral therapy, help a client recognize how their own cognitions are distorted by identifying the types of words and phrasing they use to describe their experiences. Decades of research have shown that linguistic choices have consequences on thoughts and behaviors. One well-studied type of linguistic choice and its effects on thought and behavior is generic language. A statement is generic if it is a generalization about the members of a kind or category, such as "dogs are friendly" [CARLSON1995]. Generics can also be applied to a single person. For example, "Susie is good at math, or Susie is a good drawer" reflects a general regularity about Susie compared to a nongeneric phrase of an episode such as "Susie did well on the math test today" or "Susie did a good job on her drawing" [CARLSON1995]. Research on the semantics and structure of generics suggests that they require little evidence to be taken as true, but they have strong implications because they become applied to entire categories [CIMPIAN2007].

Generic language has been found to be a common way adults use to educate children with conceptual knowledge about the world [GELMAN2004; GELMAN1998]. Concepts are similar to categories in that they help organize inputs. Some theorists propose that concepts correspond to categories, such as dogs or chairs [MARGOLIS1994]. Other theorists broaden the idea of concept to include properties (silly, tall), events or states (drawing, hurt), individuals (Mommy, Santa Claus), and abstract ideas (freedom, morality) [GELMAN2009; MEDIN2000]. When it comes to children learning concepts and adopting attitudes and behaviors to navigate an overwhelming world of stimuli, generics can be used as an efficient way of transmitting ideas. This efficiency for idea transmission is an aspect of essentialism [GELMAN2013]. Essentialism is the implicit belief that certain categories are discovered in nature and have an essential nature to them that is inherent [GELMAN2003; MEDIN1989]. The essentialist nature of generic language offers a way to simplify the world into concepts for teaching children. For example, when people hear generics about a category, such as "zarpies hate ice cream," they perceive that feature or trait to be inherent or intrinsic to that entire category more so than when they hear the same information in nongeneric form, such as "this zarpie hates ice cream" [GELMAN2010].

While using generic language is an efficient and effective way of transmitting categorical and generalizable information, this same linguistic structure also has an element of rigidity to it. In alignment with that, various cognitive therapies, as well as research on motivation and helplessness, suggest that generic language can negatively impact behavior. For example, the use of generic versus nongeneric language has been shown to influence children's post-mistake attitudes and behaviors of helplessness or mastery [CIMPIAN2007]. Another example of this comes from studies on person praise versus process praise by Carol Dweck and colleagues. They have found that when students are praised in a more essentialist way, such as "you are a good boy/girl," this fosters helpless responses after they make a mistake, in contrast to students who receive praise for their process, such as "you found a good way to do it" [KAMINS1999].

Self-Disclosure and Attributions

Another aspect of interpersonal communication that can influence people's perception of others and relationship dynamics is self-disclosure. People offer information about themselves through various verbal and nonverbal means. For example, wearing the jersey of a favorite hockey team can convey information about a person's interests in sports and particular teams. Wearing a certain style of fashion or hairstyle can convey information about a person's possible social groups. Self-disclosure is a purposeful and verbal form of offering personal information to another person. Related to self-disclosure is social penetration theory, which states that as a relationship develops, each person engages in a reciprocal process of self-disclosure and that the levels of breadth and depth of self-disclosure affect the development of the relationship [UMN2013]. Depth is related to how personal or sensitive the information is, and breadth is about the range of topics [GREENE2006]. Self-disclosure also relates to how we perceive another person based on the attributions we make about their self-disclosure. These attributions may be dispositional, situational, or interpersonal [JIANG2011]. For example, if a co-worker shares a personal detail about another co-worker, a dispositional attribution would be thinking that the reason they shared that information is due to an inherent personality trait, such as being a people-pleaser, outgoing or inappropriate [JIANG2011; UMN2013]. A situational attribution would be attributing their disclosure to context or surroundings, such as them sharing the information because another person did so. An interpersonal attribution is about the nature of the relationship. In this example, an interpersonal attribution would be if the receiver of the information believes that the fact that they are best friends with that co-worker is the reason they shared that information [JIANG2011; UMN2013]. If the receiver's main attribution is interpersonal, there is a higher chance that relational intimacy will be increased or reinforced compared to a situational or dispositional attribution for sharing the information [UMN2013]. Self-disclosure has also been found to have physical and mental health effects. Spouses of suicide or accidental health victims who did not share information with their friends have been found to have more health problems and experience more intrusive thoughts about death compared to spouses who disclosed information to friends [GREENE2006].

SUMMARY

SU, EF, and regulatory and cognitive flexibility are pillars of adaptive and effective communication due to their role in feedback responsiveness, complex perspective-taking, and language development. As we have seen in this chapter and previous ones, these pillars emerge through developmental processes over time and are therefore intrinsically connected to the journey of brain maturation, particularly in terms of prefrontal cortex development. The degree of flexibility and attunement of behavioral responses, and nuancing of language and nonverbal forms of communication in our social surroundings influences the development of neural and behavioral resources needed to foster these pillars of communication. How we use language, both internally to ourselves and with others, is influenced by and influences our evaluations of people and events. The bidirectional and complex feedback processes of communication, behavior, and how we regulate ourselves, achieving higher levels of well-being and resilience, are what we will explore further in Chapter 9.

REFERENCES

[ASTINGTON2005] Astington, J. W., and Baird, J. A. (2005). *Why Language Matters for Theory of Mind*. Oxford, UK: Oxford University Press.

[BALL2003] Ball, Robert (2003). *The Fundamentals of Aircraft Combat Survivability Analysis and Design* (2nd ed. AIAA Education Series. pp. 2, 445, 603, Reston, VA: American Institute of Aeronautics and Astronautics, Inc.

[BECK2011] Beck, JS (2011). *Cognitive Behavior Therapy: Basics and Beyond* (2nd ed.), New York, NY: The Guilford Press

[BLACKLEDGE2003] Blackledge, John T. (2003). An introduction to relational frame theory: basics and applications. *The Behavior Analyst Today*, 3, 421–433.

[BRITANNICA2016] Britannica, The Editors of Encyclopaedia. "associative learning". *Encyclopedia Britannica*, 10 June 2016, *https://www.britannica.com/topic/associative-learning*. Accessed 18 May 2023.

[CARLSON1995] Carlson, G. N., and Pelletier, F. J. (1995). *The Generic Book*. Chicago: Chicago University Press.

[CARLSON2004] Carlson, S. M., Mandell, D. J., and Williams, L. (2004). Executive function and theory of mind: Stability and prediction from age 2 to 3. *Developmental Psychology, 40*, 1105–1122.

[CHEN2014] Chen Q, et al. (2014). Association of creative achievement with cognitive flexibility by a combined voxel-based morphometry and resting-state functional connectivity study. *NeuroImage, 102*, 474–483.

[CIMPIAN2007] Cimpian, A., Arce, H. C., Markman, E. M., and Dweck, C. S. (2007). Subtle linguistic cues affect children's motivation. *Psychological Science, (1)*, 314–316.

[CLARK1998] Clark, A. (1998). Magic words: How language augments human cognition. In P. Carruthers and J. Boucher (eds.), *Language and Thought: Interdisciplinary Themes* (pp. 162–183). Cambridge: Cambridge University Press.

[CLARK2006] Clark, A. (2006). Language, embodiment, and the cognitive niche. *Trends in Cognitive Sciences, 10*, 370–374.

[CUTTING1999] Cutting, A. L., and Dunn, J. (1999). Theory of mind, emotion understanding, language, and family background: Individual differences and interrelations. *Child Development*, 70, 853–865.

[DAJANI2105] Dajani, D. R., and Uddin, L. Q. (2015). Demystifying cognitive flexibility: Implications for clinical and developmental neuroscience. *Trends in Neurosciences*, 38(9), 571–578.

[DAVIS2010] Davis, J. C., et al. (2010). The independent contribution of executive functions to health related quality of life in older women. *BMC Geriatrics, 10*,16.

[DEABREU2014] de Abreu, P. M. E., et al. (2014). Executive functioning and reading achievement in school: a study of Brazilian children assessed by their teachers as "poor readers" *Frontiers in Psychology*, 5, p. 550.

[DEVILLIERS2000] de Villiers, J. (2000). Language and theory of mind: What are the developmental relationships? In S. Baron-Cohen,

H. Tager-Flusberg, and D. J. Cohen (eds.), *Understanding Other Minds: Perspectives From Autism and Developmental Cognitive Neuroscience*. Oxford: Oxford University Press.

[DIAMOND1991] Diamond, A. (1991). Neuropsychological insights into the meaning of object concept development. In S. Carey and R. Gelman (eds.), *The Epigenesis of Mind: Essays on biology and Cognition* (pp. 67–110). Hillsdale, NJ: Erlbaum.

[DOAN2010] Doan, S. N., and Wang, Q. (2010) Maternal discussions of mental states and behaviors: relations to emotion situation knowledge in European American and immigrant Chinese children. *Child Development, 81*(5), 1490–503.

[DUNN1991] Dunn, J., Brown, J., Slomkowski, C., Tesla, C., and Youngblade, L.(1991). Young children's understanding of other people's feelings and beliefs: individual differences and their antecedents. *Child Development, 62*(6), 1352–1366.

[FAHY2014] Language and Executive Functions: Self-Talk for Self-Regulation (2014). *Perspectives on Language Learning and Education, 21*(2), 61.

[FERNYHOUGH2008] Fernyhough, C. (2008). Getting Vygotskian about theory of mind : Mediation, dialogue, and the development of social understanding. *Developmental Review, 28*(2), 225–262.

[FERNYHOUGH2010] Fernyhough, C. (2010). Vygotsky, Luria, and the social brain. In B. W. Sokol, U. Müller, J. I. M. Carpendale, A. R. Young, and G. Iarocci (Eds.), *Self and Social Regulation: Social Interaction and the Development of Social Understanding and Executive Functions* (pp. 56–79). Oxford England: Oxford University Press.

[FERNYHOUGH1996] Fernyhough, C. (1996). The dialogic mind: A dialogic approach to the higher mental functions. *New Ideas in Psychology, 14*, 47–62.

[FRAUENGLASS1985] Frauenglass, M. H., and Diaz, R. M. (1985). Self-regulatory functions of children's private speech: A critical analysis of recent challenges to Vygotsky's theory. *Developmental Psychology, 21*, 357–364.

[GELMAN1998] Gelman, S. A., Coley, J. D., Rosengren, K. S., Hartman, E., and Pappas, A. (1998). Beyond labeling: The role of parental input in the acquisition of richly-structured categories. *Monographs of the Society for Research in Child Development, 63*(1), i–148.

[GELMAN2003] Gelman, S. A. (2003). *The Essential Child: Origins of Essentialism in Everyday Thought*. New York: Oxford University Press.

[GELMAN2004] Gelman, S. A. (2004). Learning words for kinds: Generic noun phrases in acquisition. In D. G. Hall and S. R. Waxman (eds.), *Weaving a Lexicon* (pp. 445–484). Cambridge, MA: MIT Press.

[GELMAN2009] Gelman, S. A. (2009). Learning from others: Children's construction of concepts. *Annual Review of Psychology, 60:*, 15–140.

[GELMAN2010] Gelman, S. A., Ware, E., and Kleinberg, F. (2010). Effects of generic language on category content and structure. *Cognitive Psychology, 61,* 273–301.

[GELMAN2014]Gelman, S. A., Ware, E. A., Kleinberg, F., Manczak, E. M., and Stilwell, M. (2014) Individual differences in children's and parents' generic language. *Child Development*. 85(3) 924-940.

[GENET2011] Genet, J. J., and Siemer, M. (2011). Flexible control in processing affective and non-affective material predicts individual differences in trait resilience. *Cognition and Emotion, 25,* 380–388.

[GREENE2006] Greene, K., Valerian, J. Derlega, and Alicia Mathews. (2006). "Self-Disclosure in Personal Relationships," in *The Cambridge Handbook of Personal Relationships*, Anita L. Vangelisti and Daniel Perlman (eds.) (pp. 412–413). Cambridge: Cambridge University Press.

[HARRIS1999] Harris, P. L. (1999). Acquiring the art of conversation. In M. Bennett (ed.), *Developmental Psychology: Achievements and Prospects* (pp. 89–105). Hove, UK: Psychology Press.

[HAYES2001] Hayes, S. C., Barnes-Holmes, D., and Roche, B. (2001). *Relational Frame Theory: A Post-Skinnerian Account of Human Language and Cognition*. New York: Kluwer Academic/Plenum Publishers.

[HERMER1999] Hermer-Vazquez, L., Spelke, E. S., and Katsnelson, A. S. (1999). Sources of flexibility in human cognition: Dual-task studies of space and language. *Cognitive Psychology, (39),* 1.

[HUGHES2005] Hughes, C., and Ensor, R. (2005). Executive function and theory of mind in 2 year olds: A family affair? *Developmental Neuropsychology, 28,* 645–668.

[JENKINS1996] Jenkins, J. M., and Astington, J. W. (1996). Cognitive factors and family structure associated with theory of mind development in young children. *Developmental Psychology, 32,* 70–78.

[JIANG2011] Jiang, L. C., Natalie N. Bazarova, and Jeffrey T. Hancock (2011). The disclosure-intimacy link in computer-mediated communication: An attributional extension of the hyperpersonal model. *Human Communication Research, 37,* 63.

[KAMINS1999] Kamins, M., and Dweck, C. S. (1999). Person vs. process praise and criticism: Implications for contingent self-worth and coping. *Developmental Psychology, 35,* 835–847.

[KOHLBERG1968] Kohlberg, L., Yaeger, J., and Hjertholm, E. (1968). Private speech: Four studies and a review of theories. *Child Development, 39,* 691–736.

[LEWIS1996] Lewis C, Freeman NH, Kyriakidou C, Maridaki-Kassotaki K, Berridge DM. (1996). Social influences on false belief access: specific sibling influences or general apprenticeship? *Child Development, 67*(6), 2930–2947.

[LURIA1965] Luria, A.R. (1965). L. S. Vygotsky and the problem of localization of functions. *Neuropsychologia, (3),* 387–392.

[MALKINSON2013] Malkinson, R., and Brask-Rustad, T. (2013). Cognitive behavior couple therapy-REBT model for traumatic bereavement. *Journal of Rational-Emotive and Cognitive-Behavior Therapy, 31*(2), 114–125.

[MARGOLIS1994] Margolis, E. (1994). A reassessment of the shift from the classical theory of concepts to prototype theory. *Cognition (51),* 73–89.

[MEDIN1989] Medin, D. L. (1989). Concepts and conceptual structure. *American Psychologist, (44),* 1469–1481.

[MEDIN2000] Medin, D. L., Lynch, E. B., and Solomon, K. O. (2000) Are there kinds of concepts? *Annual Review of Psychology, 51,* 121–47.

[MEAD1934] Mead, G. H. (1934). *Mind, Self and Society From the Standpoint of a Social Behaviorist.* Chicago: University of Chicago Press.

[MEINS1998] Meins, E., Fernyhough, C., Russell, J., and Clark-Carter, D. (1998). Security of attachment as a predictor of symbolic and mentalising abilities: A longitudinal study. *Social Development, 7,* 1–24.

[MEINS2002] Meins, E., Fernyhough, C., Wainwright, R., Das Gupta, M., Fradley, E., and Tuckey, M. (2002). Maternal mind-mindedness and attachment security as predictors of theory of mind understanding.. *Child Development, 73,* 1715–1726.

[MULLER2004] Müller, U., Zelazo, P. D., Hood, S., Leone, T., and Rohrer, L. (2004). Interference control The social brain 35 in a new rule use task: Age-related changes, labeling, and attention. *Child Development, 75,* 1594–1609.

[OLTEAN2017] Oltean, H. R., Hyland, P., Vallieres, F., and David, D. O. (2017). An empirical assessment of REBT models of psychopathology and psychological health in the prediction of anxiety and depression symptoms. *Behavioral and Cognitive Psychotherapy, 45*(6), 600–615.

[PERNER2002] Perner, J., Lang, B., and Kloo, D. (2002). Theory of mind and self-control: More than a common problem of inhibition. *Child Development, 73,* 752–767.

[UMN2013] University of Minnesota Publishing *Communication in the Real World: An Introduction to Communication Studies* is adapted from a work produced and distributed under a Creative Commons license (CC BY-NC-SA) in 2013 by a publisher who has requested that they and the original author not receive attribution.

[VYGOTSKY1978] Vygotsky, L. S. (1978). *Mind in Society: The Development of Higher Mental Processes*, M. Cole, V. John-Steiner, S. Scribner, and E. Souberman (eds. and trans.). Cambridge, MA: Harvard University Press. (Original work published 1930–1935).

[VYGOTSKY1987] Vygotsky, L. S. (1987). Thinking and speech. *In the Collected Works of L. S. Vygotsky, Vol. 1.* New York: Plenum. (Original work published 1934).

[WERTSCH1985] Wertsch, J. V. (1985). *Vygotsky and the social formation of mind.* Cambridge, MA: Harvard University Press.

[WINSLER1997] Winsler, A., Diaz, R. M., and Montero, I. (1997). The role of private speech in the transition from collaborative to independent task performance in young children. *Early Childhood Research Quarterly, 12,* 59–79.

[WINSLER2003] Winsler, A., and Naglieri, J. (2003). Overt and covert verbal problem-solving strategies: Developmental trends in use, awareness, and Relations with Task Performance in Children Aged 5 to 17, *Child Development (74)*, 3: 659-678.

[WINSLER2004] Winsler, A. (2004). Still talking to ourselves after all these years: Vygotsky, private speech, and self-regulation. Invited address given at First International Symposium on Self-Regulatory Functions of Language, Madrid, November 2004.

[WINSLER?] Winsler, A., Fernyhough, C., and Montero, I. (forthcoming). *Private Speech, Executive Functioning, and the Development of Verbal Self-regulation.* Cambridge, UK: Cambridge University Press.

[WINSLER2009] Winsler, A. (2009). Still talking to ourselves after all these years: A Review of current research on private speech. In *Private Speech, Executive Functioning, and the Development of Verbal Self-Regulation* (pp. 3-41). A. Winsler, C. Fernyhough, and I. Montero (eds.). Cambridge: Cambridge University Press.

[ZETTLE2016] Zettle, R. D., Hayes, S. C., Barnes-Holmes, D., and Biglan, A. (2016). *The Wiley Handbook of Contextual Behavioral Science* (pp. 28–68). Oxford, UK: Wiley.

SYSTEMS RESILIENCE

What does it mean to survive? Is there a difference between survival and resilience? What makes a person, community, or relationship capable of withstanding setbacks, tragedies, and disruptions? How can we learn from systems engineering and the concept of resilience from other disciplines to inspire and innovate new ways to approach human well-being? In previous chapters, we looked at how regulatory flexibility plays a role in our ability to communicate and achieve an overall goal of systems regulation. We also explored nonverbal and verbal communication as a mechanism for homeostasis and looked at how our social experiences impact brain networks, cognitive processing, and executive functioning, as well as internally and externally focused speech. We will now look at how all of these are integrated into an overall framework of systems resilience. In this chapter, we will return to our question: what is communication for? With this in mind, we understand that communication is a *tool* and a technology, and it serves as a mechanism to support the overarching goal of every dynamic system: to survive. As we think about survival, we need to keep in mind that this encompasses both maintenance of internal systems and recovery, as well as projection into the future. To achieve this goal, a system must be resilient. This is true whether we are thinking of a human as a system, a family, a community, a country, or even artificial intelligence systems. Communication is feedback and feedback is the essential component to all aspects of resilience, complexity, and survivability. Communication is therefore a tool or technology for ensuring systems resilience.

The idea of resilience has increasingly emerged in research over recent years due to its role in reducing the risks that can come from the inevitable disruption of systems [HOSSEINI2016]. The term resilience essentially means to "bounce back," and resilience researchers propose a variety of definitions that include words like robustness, survivability, and agility [HOSSEINI 2016]. An important element that is also often included in resilience is preparedness and anticipation, as well as mitigating, responding, and recovering from adverse conditions and events [CARLSON2012]. A full, holistic approach to resilience includes all of these elements. We will see later in this chapter how resilience engineering concepts relate to interpersonal communication ideas such as rupture and repair. First, we will take an overall view of systems resilience.

RESILIENCE AND SURVIVABILITY

As we explore a systems resilience approach to understanding communication, the military definition of survivability offers useful parallels. Resilience is often used interchangeably with the concept of survivability; however, the military definition of survivability also includes the ability of the system to remain "mission capable" after an engagement [BALL2003]. This component of remaining mission capable relates to a complex system's way of thinking. As discussed in earlier chapters, to truly understand if a system, strategy, or mechanism is performing well, we must understand its purpose. If we do not think about its overall mission and function, we may isolate components or analyze outcomes that do not serve or reflect the system's highest level of functioning [ACKOFF1994]. An analogy of this offered by the late systems analyst Russell Ackoff is a car. A car is a system. It has an overall function of moving a person from one location to another. Because we understand what it is for,[1] we can then explore how to measure its operations in terms of effectiveness (is it doing what it is supposed to be doing?) and efficiency (is it using the least amount of energy possible to perform at its highest capacity based on the architecture and environment?). The mission-capable approach to maintaining, operating, and improving a car keeps the mission in mind and views all components as subsystems that perform this mission together in ways that are impossible for each component to do by itself. The engine, by itself, cannot transport a person. The wheels, by themselves, cannot transport a person (although they roll, you would still need another mechanism to keep them in a formation that would synchronize their movement to keep a person stable on top and moving in a streamlined direction). It is only when all components come together to perform their function toward a *unified* mission that they become a system [ACKOFF1994]. Otherwise, they are just isolated parts.

---

[1] On a certain level. There are deeper philosophical levels we could also consider, such as, why do we want to move efficiently from one location to another, but that's for another book).

To analyze whether each component is functioning at its highest capacity, we must take the overall, unified mission of the car into consideration. Measuring air pressure and texture of a tire and rolling it by itself gives us some information about the tire. Yet this alone cannot tell us if it will enhance the overall mission of the car. Too much pressure in a tire may not serve the purpose of a vehicle that is designed for certain terrains and maneuvers but will be optimal for other types of terrains and maneuvers. The mission or purpose of the vehicle is a key part of what allows us to truly know if the strategies and tools we are using to enhance each component are doing what we need them to do.

The military definition of survivability is therefore an integral part of systems resilience. When we talk about communication, what system are we considering it to be a part of? One person alone is a component of a larger system such as that of a relationship, dyad, group, community, or species. Because of the hyper-connectedness of the human species, particularly as it relates to our current phase of evolution and technological capability of communicating on global scale, the idea of communication when it comes to humans must include a species-wide perspective. As we have seen repeatedly throughout this book, our social experiences are conveyed through signals and frequencies that we project out and detect from others. Those signals and frequencies have direct effects on our internal experiences and neural network activity. The communication that occurs between two people or "nodes" has effects on each person's nervous system and the subsequent behaviors, thoughts, internal states, and attitudes they will adopt in response to the signals they have transmitted and received during that interaction. Those behaviors, thoughts, internal states, and attitudes will play a role in that person's subsequent communication with another person (online and in person). Moreover, as we have already discussed, the goal of any living system is homeostasis (more technically speaking, to resist entropy). Homeostasis includes both maintenance of physical integrity and internal systems, as well as an ability to project into the future. Communication is one of the mechanisms we use as humans to achieve our goal of homeostasis. Keeping all of this in mind, this final chapter will highlight some key principles of systems resilience as a pillar of human species survivability and the role of communication as a tool for enhancing systems resilience.

To do this, we will first explore the paradigm of networks and systems resilience from an engineering perspective. We will then move back into our previously explored frameworks for human communication and resilience from the perspective of regulatory flexibility and feedback responsiveness.

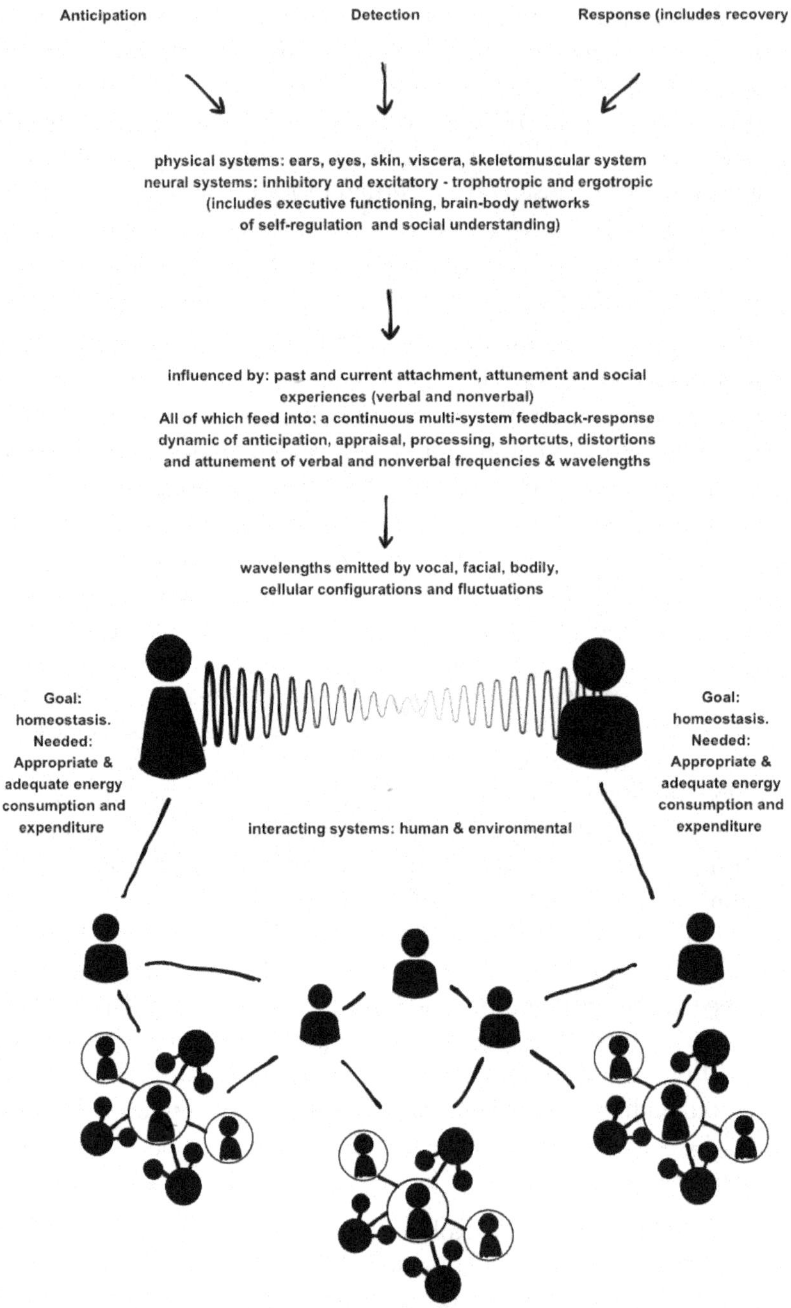

Anticipation   Detection   Response (includes recovery

physical systems: ears, eyes, skin, viscera, skeletomuscular system
neural systems: inhibitory and excitatory - trophotropic and ergotropic
(includes executive functioning, brain-body networks
of self-regulation and social understanding)

influenced by: past and current attachment, attunement and social
experiences (verbal and nonverbal)
All of which feed into: a continuous multi-system feedback-response
dynamic of anticipation, appraisal, processing, shortcuts, distortions
and attunement of verbal and nonverbal frequencies & wavelengths

wavelengths emitted by vocal, facial, bodily,
cellular configurations and fluctuations

Goal: Goal:
homeostasis.   homeostasis.
Needed: Needed:
Appropriate &   Appropriate &
adequate energy   adequate energy
consumption and   consumption and
expenditure   interacting systems: human & environmental   expenditure

FIGURE 9.1 Systems resilience overview of human communication.

WHAT MAKES A SYSTEM RESILIENT?

Keeping the military definition of survivability as a foundation for resilience, a system is resilient if it is able to carry out its mission despite disruptions, excessive stressors, threats, and other challenges [FIRESMITH2003]. These adversities could be caused by a variety of factors, including [FIRESMITH2020]:

1. Defects in the architecture (hardware and software) of the system. An example of issues with hardware in humans would be genetic or developmental disruptions and disorders. Software is inputted into a system, so defects in this could include negligent or maladaptive communication and attunement from caregivers.

2. Lack of safeguards to prevent accidents and trauma. This may include preventive measures such as nutrition, sleep, and safeguards for physical trauma such as how protected a home is against environmental conditions or danger. Trauma is related to allostatic load, which is when an event or conditions exceed the neural and behavioral resources and capacities of a person, which can lead to a bias of energy over-expenditure or under-expenditure through trophotropic or ergotropic responses (see Chapter 2).

3. External environmental conditions. For humans, this may include things like noise levels in the home or community, physical safety in the home or community, as well as events like natural disasters, unrest, and violence.

Some definitions of systems resilience also include the avoidance of adverse events and conditions [BRTIS2019]. According to other engineering experts, however, avoiding or preventing adversities does not make a system more resilient [HOSSEINI2016; FIRESMITH2020]. Conversely, avoiding adversity decreases the need for system resilience and, therefore, does not push the system to adopt what is needed to become resilient [FIRESMITH2020]. Therefore, a more advanced definition of systems resilience includes the idea that a system will inevitably face adverse events and conditions. The defining questions for understanding a system's resilience are about how the system detects, responds, and recovers from adverse events and conditions. To truly know the resilience of a system, we must know its capability to continue to carry out its function despite potentially suboptimal conditions, disturbances, adversities, and degraded or weakened states [FIRESMITH2020]. Moreover, it must be able to recover quickly from any damage that may have occurred.

Passive and Active Resilience

To do this, two types of resilience are needed: active and passive resilience [FIRESMITH2020]. Active system resilience involves the detection of threats and adversity, the ability to react accordingly, and the ability to recover. Passive system resilience includes anticipation that adverse conditions and events are inevitable and building in a high level of capacity and redundancies to help the system resist or avoid disruptions. An example using a car would be adding reinforcement, such as a brush or deer guard, to the front of the vehicle, if the car is being driven in areas where there may be wildlife to prevent damage that could disrupt the capabilities of the vehicle. In humans, this could include nutrition, exercise, sleep, and preventive types of therapy to increase the capacity of the person to withstand stressors. While these may not seem to be related to communication, they all play a role in the internal state and the neural resources available to a person at any given moment. This in turn impacts the signals they are transmitting as well as how they perceive and process the signals sent by others during communicative interactions. If someone has not slept well, is hungry, ill, or in mental distress, they will detect and project micro-expressions, words, and behaviors differently than when they are well-rested and in good overall health. It is these types of factors that comprise a systems thinking and systems resilience perspective when we cover a topic such as communication. It is not just about the words, or facial gestures. It is not just about one person. It is about all the factors that go into each moment that we interact with others. Those moments are consequences of the various systems, subsystems, and events that have led up to or are still currently influencing the functioning of each person. Understanding this reveals how deeply intertwined communication is with mental and physical health, and many other dimensions of human experience. This wider-system view can also help us explore many possibilities for improving the effectiveness of communication so that we can use it for its purpose of optimizing our functioning and survivability.

A resilient system is capable of protecting its critical capabilities in order to keep fulfilling its mission. It uses passive techniques to help it resist threats and harm, as well as active techniques to detect, respond to, and recover from adversity. Communication, as we have seen in previous chapters, is implicated in many of these strategies. The feedback aspect of communication, particularly when we are little, plays a major role in building the neural architecture needed for self-regulation, social understanding, and executive function. The nonverbal communication that occurs in our social experiences influences our internal states and behaviors that serve to either protect us from threats or take advantage of opportunities. Verbal communication elements contribute to internal dialogues that help us solve problems and lay a foundation for how we feel and think about ourselves, which in turn contributes to how we are able to cope with things like social rejection or challenging social interactions. The communication that occurs between caregivers and children plays a significant role in the child's perception and processing of input from emotional expressions and words of others, which feeds into their regulatory flexibility and ability to use adequate and adaptive responses to what is occurring.

Many of these features overlap with concepts related to systems resilience from an engineering perspective. These concepts include protecting critical capabilities and assets, resisting adverse events and conditions, detecting, reacting to, and recovering from adversities and disturbances. In the next section, we will look at some of these concepts and how they overlap with elements of human communication.

PROTECTION

A system's ability to protect itself relies on the following four elements: resistance, detection, reaction, and recovery.

Resistance: In systems engineering, *resistance* can include architecture that is made up of modules to prevent failure propagation and lack of single points of failure, and protective shielding of equipment from electromagnetic pulses [FIRESMITH2019]. The main principle is that these are introduced to a system as a way to passively prevent or minimize harm from adverse events or conditions. In the realm of human communication, we can see this principle in terms of self-regulating architecture in the prefrontal cortex developing through nonverbal and verbal feedback from social interactions so that a person can eventually regulate their own system even if another person is unavailable or unable to. The mechanism developed through evolution to help us protect ourselves lies in this self-regulating dimension. The degree of how well these self-regulating abilities protect us from harm are influenced by our experiences. The stronger our executive functioning and self-regulating architecture become, the more we are able to accurately perceive threats and opportunities and flexibly respond to them using our resources efficiently and effectively.

Detection: To protect itself, a system must also be able to *detect* the following [FIRESMITH2019]:

- Loss or harm of its capabilities.

- Damage to assets that are needed to implement those capabilities.

- Adverse events or conditions that could cause disturbances or harm to those capabilities or assets. Adverse events or conditions include environmental events, input or operator errors, accidents, attacks, excessive loads, excessive wear and tear, external conditions that exceed the system's tolerance and capacities, system-internal faults such as hardware-software defects, lack of safety, loss of or degraded communications (interoperability), vulnerabilities to attack and damage.

Detection techniques for harm, damage, and adversity in humans are related to our five senses in conjunction with our interoceptive abilities. Our ability to detect danger or threat in the realm of human communication and interaction includes seeing facial expressions, hearing voice frequencies, detecting other subtle frequencies such as smell, pupil dilation, how the person is breathing, body posture movements, and verbal signals that could indicate a person's internal state or intention as something that could harm us. Detecting these using the senses is integrated with our interoceptive abilities: this is our ability to sense how our internal state and organs such as heart and skin are responding to stimuli. These visceral sensations travel up to the brain to give it data to process for how to respond and communicate. As we saw in the Component Process Model for emotions (Chapter 5), the affective state we experience in response to input is tied to our perceived ability to cope and whether we perceive something as an obstacle to a goal [SCHERER2013]. We also saw in the dynamic maturational model (Chapter 4) that our processing of information may distort how we are perceiving social and emotional cues from others. This would be an example of input or operator errors. Our attentional biases may also hone our attention on specific features or words of an interaction that may distort our perception. This means that although we have detection techniques to protect us from harm, there are many complex processes that also influence our perception of threats. The more flexible and self-regulating we become, using feedback responsiveness to make adjustments as needed, we can improve the accuracy of our detection techniques. This is due to the fact that dysregulation may narrow our attention excessively onto certain features of a person or scene [FREDERIKSON2005], which may then limit the overall context and other information that could determine if something is actually a threat or not. An example would be noticing (detecting) a frown on someone's face and reacting immediately as though they were angry, without opening one's awareness to other factors, such as the possibility that an upsetting event had just occurred or that they are holding a sympathy card in their hand. On the flip side, detecting an unusual pattern in someone's behavior and having a "gut feeling" that something is wrong and acting accordingly is a detection technique that protects us from harm. The more open, accurate, and present-moment a person's detection abilities are, the more context-sensitive and adaptive their response will be because it is interacting with actually occurring input (rather than distorted or narrowed attention). Although systems engineering generally refers to detection in the context of threat, in terms of human communication, detection can also be used to accurately perceive situations as opportunities to gain beneficial resources in some form, including social support, co-regulation, networking, etc.

Reaction: In addition to being able to protect against and detect adversities, systems resilience also includes a system's ability to *react* to an ongoing or emerging adversity. In response to a challenge, a system might attempt to stop the event or remove the adverse condition as a way of minimizing further disruption or degradation [FIRESMITH2019]. The parallel in human communication is the concept of feedback responsiveness discussed in Chapter 3. As a quick review, feedback responsiveness includes the willingness and ability to increase, change, or cease a strategy according to live, ongoing, and emerging feedback. If communication is meant to be a tool for enhancing systems resilience, one of the key pillars for effective communication is feedback responsiveness. This is in contrast to repeatedly using the same types of words, tone, gestures, and other nonverbal or verbal cues within an interaction, regardless of what feedback is coming back. Effective reactions include flexibility of response. This would mean that if a person began a conversation with angry words and tone but received feedback (the other person's words and tone) that added new information or context, then feedback responsiveness would mean an adjustment of verbal and nonverbal information in response to the new and emerging data, rather than their original mood, view, or reaction. The types of reactions to perceived threat in human communication tie into accurately detecting actual-physical threat versus social threats and are also tied to the person's existing biases toward noticing and interpreting facial expressions based on past experiences.

Recovery: In order to truly protect the integrity of a system's capabilities and mission, various strategies need to be in place before a threat occurs in order to resist and detect the adversity, as well as an ability to react during the challenge and finally also an ability to recover from any harm or disturbance caused by the adverse event or condition. From a systems resilience perspective, recovery may be complete, partial, or minimal [FIRESMITH2019]. Complete recovery means that any damage that occurred has been repaired or replaced, and the system is once again operating at full capacity. Partial recovery means some of the damage was not replaced or repaired, but the system has returned to full functioning using redundant resources [FIRESMITH2019]. Recovery is minimal when the system is not fully functional again and operating with limited capacity. Recovery can also include the entire system reconfiguring itself in order to evolve or adapt to future occurrences of adversities [FIRESMITH2019]. The idea of recovery parallels the concept of rupture and repair, which is a foundation of the child-caregiver dynamic for building self-regulatory neural and behavioral resources and is also a foundation for secure attachment in adult relationships.

RUPTURE, REPAIR, AND FLEXIBLE RESPONSIVENESS

Because self-regulatory systems are not ready-made at birth, human caregiver–child interactions include the major task of building these systems. As we have seen from a system's optimization viewpoint, *flexibility* is key. Flexible responsiveness—the ability to constantly adapt, cease, increase, or change strategies according to continuously emerging and dynamic inputs—holds the key to not only survival but also optimization of energy use for future projection. To build this flexibility, the task of a caregiver is to help build tolerance and a large repertoire of strategies for the child to modulate their internal state and tolerate a variety of levels of arousal. The wider the range of these internal states, the more the child will develop neural and behavioral resources to adapt and modify accordingly. The narrower the range of internal states, the fewer networks and strategies the brain needs to use energy to build. Because the brain-body system is an energy-conserving system, it only devotes resources to what is called upon by the environment. This is a key element of experience-dependent brain development, which we first discussed in Chapter 1. Therefore, introducing a child to a large variety of states of arousal is a caregiving strategy for helping build sophisticated self-regulatory systems within the child's brain-body system. One mechanism for doing this is the distress-relief or rupture-repair sequence [SCHORE1994]. We saw a few arousal modulation strategies between caregiver and child in Chapter 2, where we discussed eye gaze, and the excitatory arousal levels it causes in the infant. We then saw that intrusive caregiving means that the caregiver continues to attempt to prolong the excitatory state in the child through voice, facial expression, and movement and does not attune to the child's signal that it is attempting to downregulate its own state by averting the caregiver's gaze. In attuned arousal modulation, the caregiver uses face, voice, eyes, and movement to engage the child's attention and induce a higher positive arousal state, and then tunes into cues from the child that they have reached a level beyond their own internal capacity to regulate, triggering a sequence of behaviors that dampen the arousal level, such as mirroring the averted gaze, quieting the voice, and flattening facial expression. This same type of arousal modulation is also with the rupture-repair framework. For low levels of distress, the child may be able to use their own self-regulatory systems. In many cases, however, the distress of the child requires active modulation from the caregiver [SCHORE1994]. In order to help build the child's systems for higher levels of negative arousal and distress, the caregiver uses strategies that are misattuned to the child's signals. If the child is in an excitatory or exploratory mode, the caregiver will use a facial expression or voice of disapproval to minimize and dampen the child's ever-increasing hyperarousal. This strategy enables the child to experience a high level of positive arousal, followed by an abrupt dampening of arousal as a way to build internal nervous system mechanisms to minimize uninhibited or unsafe exploratory and excitatory behaviors [SCHORE1994]. The goal of the caregiver is not to maintain a constant positive arousal or calm regulated state in the child but rather to help the child experience a wide range of internal and visceral states with sequences of behaviors that can modulate those states.

Rupture and repair strategies have also been studied in adult relationships, particularly married couples. In a microanalytic coding system of couples' communicative strategies, the Couples Interactions Scoring System (CISS), couples high in marital satisfaction have reported higher mutuality, while couples lower in marital satisfaction report higher levels of destructive process, coercion, and postconflict distress [JULIEN1989; GOTTMAN2001]. Coding of facial expressions has also led to coding systems that reveal patterns of marital interaction during both conflict and nonconflict contexts. These studies include coding from the Marital Interaction Coding System [WEISS1990], the Emotion Facial Action Coding System [EKMAN1978], a rapid version of the CISS called the RCISS [KROKOFF1989], and the Specific Affect Coding System [GOTTMAN1996]. The studies integrating these coding systems have led to reliable microanalytic real-time data for marital nonverbal and verbal communication. A meta-review exploring marital conflict used these coding frameworks to organize rupture and repair strategies into a seven-stage process that begins with an event that precipitates the conflict, evolution through the conflict, and then a return to normal [CHRISTENSEN1993].

It is not the absence of conflict or disruption that predicts necessarily whether a couple will report marital satisfaction and/or remain married, but rather the types of strategies used, particularly during and after conflict. It is the *recovery* that matters. Some studies have reported a high level of accuracy in predicting divorce using coding systems that measure physiological and neural correlates of marital behaviors as they engage in problem-solving and contexts of conflict. Studies by Gottman and colleagues have found that the ratio of positivity to negativity during conflict discussion, and four specific types of negative interaction (criticism, defensiveness, contempt, and stonewalling) are highly predictive of divorce [GOTTMAN1993; 1994; 1998; MATTHEWS1996]. Effective repair attempts, on the other hand, include reducing negative affect or increasing positive affect during conflict. [GOTTMAN2015]. Pre-emptive repair, which occurs in the first 3 minutes of conflict is shown to be most effective at repair and address the affective tone of the interaction as a way to create emotional connection, rather than appeal to cognitive problem-solving or rationality [GOTTMAN2015]. Some of these affective repairs include words or gestures that indicate "we're okay," shared humor, affection, self-disclosure, expressing understanding and empathy, as well as taking responsibility for an aspect of the problem being discussed [GOTTMAN2015].

We can see from the above studies on rupture and repair in adult relationships that they mirror many aspects of the co-regulating dynamic between caregivers and child. There are components within the two-person system of a relationship, such as marriage, that engage a range and repertoire of arousal states and affect-modulation strategies, with each partner playing a role in the system's ability to regulate. When recovery techniques used by these relational systems are effective, they help free up neural and behavioral resources for problem-solving and recovery.

ASSETS

For a system to be resilient, another factor to keep in mind is not only that protection is vital, but what exactly is the system trying to protect? Within the system's resilience framework, we consider *assets* to be the items of value that are critical to carrying out the system's mission. Because assets are related to the capabilities of a system, they also therefore play an essential part in the overall goal of human communication as a tool for human system survival and optimization. Assets include system components, system data, and system-external assets [FIRESMITH2019].

System components include subsystems, hardware, networks, software, and facilities [FIRESMITH2019]. If we think of human brain-body and relational systems, these assets would be reflected in the various nervous system components, including those we explored in previous chapters, such as facial muscles, vagus nerve connections to ears, vocal muscles, heart and face, the unique human configuration for breathing and its connections to nervous system state and voice, the neural networks that get developed through experiences, particularly social experiences, and the environments we are surrounded by.

System data relates to how data is stored, produced, and manipulated [FIRESMITH2019]. We saw also in previous chapters that there are various systems involved in how the data from our physical, social, and internal environments are sensed, stored, and interpreted. For example, in Chapter 2, we looked at implicit memory and how many of the inputs we receive are stored in ways that are inaccessible to our conscious awareness but nonetheless prepare our body and attentional mechanisms to notice features of what is happening based on past experiences. We also explored the concept of subcortical shortcuts in Chapter 4, which highlighted how our brain-body systems may distort how we process information. In Chapter 7, we discussed the manipulation of internal, visceral, and sensory information into symbolic and verbal representations. System data within human communication would also include the frequencies and signals that are detected and transmitted within each social interaction.

System-external assets include people, environments, funds, and reputation [FIRESMITH2019]. These are all assets that enhance the functioning of a system. For example, a positive reputation can induce higher levels of social and financial support; highly trained and experienced people can come up with more nuanced solutions for enhancing the system's functioning. Within the context of human communication and its interplay with nervous system regulation and optimization, system-external assets would include all the various systems that intersect, overlap, and influence a person's internal state, neural activity, architecture, and reactions. These include family, community members, friends, and teachers, as well as other supports like therapy, and access to funds that can help maintain and improve basic functions through nutrition, physical safety, protection from harm, abuse and addiction, sleep, and many other external factors. Reputation is also a factor in all relational dynamics, including family systems. One member's reputation can be based on how they respond or the types of behavior they engage in and what they prioritize in terms of values and activities (e.g., do they consider only their interests, or do they value the interests and opinions of others; do they have a low tolerance for distress and often display angry outbursts). Commonly occurring behaviors and reactions may form the basis of how others will anticipate and prepare for interactions with that person. The entire family will also build a reputation within their communities and networks based on their behaviors and responses, which will also influence the amount and type of social support they may receive from people outside the family.

When we think about processes to help us improve the effectiveness of communication, we can include the idea that we must protect these assets through the strategies mentioned earlier: resistance and detection. Resistance includes building up protective mechanisms to help withstand disruptions and adversities. Detection includes finding tools and assessments that can help accurately detect when systems are functioning and when they are dysregulated—such as physiological data like heart rate variability, skin conductance, brainwaves, facial electromyography, voice frequencies, and body posture and movement.

QUALITY ATTRIBUTES OF RESILIENCE

In addition to the above-mentioned components, resilience is also influenced by quality attributes. These include the following [FIRESMITH2020]:

- Adaptability: this can include an ability to restructure, reconfigure, and balance loads differently in order to respond and recover from adversity.

- Availability: a resilient system maintains the availability of its critical capabilities even during the occurrence of adverse events or conditions.

- Maintainability and reparability: a system is more resilient if it can repair and maintain itself rather than rely on something external to do this.

- Performance: resilience strategies (detection, response, and recovery) use a lot of energy, resources, and bandwidth, which can affect real-time performance—resilient systems must strike a balance in using resources efficiently according to environmental circumstances and what is required for high levels of functioning.

- Reliability: when a system is not reliable, this leads to faults and failures, which then requires more energy resources for detection, response, and recovery.

We see the above quality attributes in the various frameworks and concepts explored throughout this book, particularly in the realm of self-regulation abilities and regulatory flexibility.

GUIDING PRINCIPLES FOR RESILIENT SYSTEMS

Below are some guiding principles suggested by systems engineering expert Donald Firesmith [FIRESMITH2020; FIRESMITH2003]:

Focus on mission-critical capabilities. This brings us back to the systems thinking perspective of what communication is for. What are we trying to do when we communicate? Exploring this way of thinking can help drill down to mission-critical capabilities. Communication is a tool or subcomponent of an overall system for achieving homeostasis. The mission of homeostasis (survival and future projection) is achieved through a regulation of nervous system activities that allow for adequate restoration and recovery for vital systems, movement of skeletal-muscular systems to protect the physical structures of the body, and efficient use of neural and sociobehavioral mechanisms for extracting resources from the environment. Communicating is a way for humans to support the capabilities of achieving that mission of homeostasis. Therefore, when we examine how to enhance these capabilities, such as how and what we say to others, it can be helpful to think about how words, voice frequencies, facial expressions, and gestures either enhance or diminish one's ability to regulate their nervous system, protect themselves from harm and achieve goals through social support. Focusing on these mission-critical capabilities may help people identify what truly needs to be expressed and what may not need to be in a given moment. The goal of systems resilience is to ensure that mission-critical capabilities are not disrupted during adverse events or conditions. How do we improve communication strategies to support this goal?

Identify critical assets. Critical assets include the system components of hardware and software, systems data, and system-external data sources. Within the realm of human communication, we see that these assets include our nervous system and how it operates, the signals and frequencies we are inputting into and receiving from social interactions, and the people and environments we are surrounded by and connected to. To enhance systems resilience, all of these assets must be identified and protected as much as possible.

Concentrate on common critical assets. These include shared networks, services, and data repositories. From a human communication perspective, this includes all social communication platforms, as well as the spaces in each person's life where people are relying on a shared source of information, which can be a platform but also a person such as a teacher, leader, or role model.

Concentrate on disruptive harm [FIRESMITH2020]. Not all conditions or events will disrupt mission-critical capabilities. Resilience engineering is about concentrating on harm that is capable of disrupting these. This aligns with the regulatory principle of context sensitivity. The better we get at discerning what factors in our physical, internal, and social environments are actual threats and which ones are potentially being distorted by our attentional biases, the better we use energy efficiently for system functioning. This also means that conditions, such as high-risk parenting, neglect, and abuse, which have been studied and validated by developmental and neurophysiological research to be detrimental to self-regulating neural architecture, are factors that do harm mission-critical capabilities and must therefore be primary focus on resilience engineering.

Expect and identify adversities [FIRESMITH2020]. Resilience engineering does not include avoidance of adversity, but rather designing strategies that assume that adverse conditions and events are a part of existence and *will* occur. This includes acknowledging many types of adversities, that multiple challenges can occur at once, and they may vary over time. Humans are complex systems with many unconscious and experience-based reactions, assumptions, and biases. To help us navigate challenges, it is important to build flexibly responsive and self-regulating networks that will enable us to navigate constantly emerging threats and opportunities. As people engage in childcare, developing family networks, education, and therapy programs, professional development, and any type of activity that is meant to help people optimize their mental health, well-being, and functioning, the acknowledgment of the inevitability of adversity can help guide resilience-enhancing activities and modeling. Moreover, a systems thinking approach to resilience acknowledges that challenges can overlap, compile, and accumulate or change over time. This means that it is important to address the many types of assets that can be affected by environmental and social inputs. For example, a lack of sleep, poor nutrition, or lack of social support may contribute to a nervous system degradation that makes it harder to self-regulate. Resilience engineering therefore must address the multiplicity of conditions and events that can degrade a system or increase vulnerability. Because there may be many adversities, it is also sometimes necessary to triage, or prioritize a subset in terms of their probability of occurrence and the level of harm they may be able to cause.

Anticipate, resist, detect, react, recover [CARLSON2012; FIRESMITH2020]. As noted earlier, some definitions of resilience focus on what happens after an adverse event occurs, while others look at factors that build resilience before the event, such as resistance, protection, anticipation, and preparedness [CARLSON2012]. The most comprehensive definitions include all of these components, both passive and active. Resistance is the passive element of resilience. This can include laying the groundwork that will help the system withstand conditions and events. Passive resistance can sometimes be more energy efficient and effective than active resistance such as detecting, reacting, and recovering from adversities; however, both passive and active techniques are needed to protect mission-critical capabilities. Because human communication relies on the internal state of each person and we know that internal experiences are influenced by distortions in human perception based on previous experiences, and unconscious processes, resilience engineering that includes passive and active techniques for self-regulation and improvement, cognitive processing is therefore a component of improving the effectiveness of communication. The following are some examples of passive and active resilience techniques that relate to human interpersonal functioning.

Anticipation and resistance acknowledge the inevitability of adverse conditions and events. Through anticipation, foresight, and preparedness, we can use past research and observations to build statistics and increase the predictive power of how things may go wrong in terms of healthy brain development and therefore optimized self-regulation and communication abilities. We see this in the field of prevention science, where, for example, social-emotional competencies are taught to parents before the birth of a child, as well as ongoing support for parents in a variety of forms. Other elements of prevention science can also include wider-systems strategies, such as integrating training and assistance for optimizing nutrition and sleep in conjunction with social-emotional and parenting training.

Detection, reaction, recovery: Detection comes in the form of assessments and check-ins to try to detect disruptions or vulnerabilities before they become bigger issues. With a deeper understanding of the biological mechanisms and manifestations of internal states and how these are expressed, detected, and processed, we can increase the sophistication of detection strategies. For example, measuring heart rate variability is a way to understand the vagal tone and vagus nerve functioning for flexibly moving across ranges of parasympathetic and sympathetic responses. Voice frequency and facial muscle analysis can contribute to an understanding of a person's internal state and abilities to express emotional tones and gestures. Self-reports and observations from others in terms of how a person is describing their experiences and how they are internally feeling can also reveal interoceptive abilities and emotional granularity. Getting an inventory of these within school, family, community, and professional settings would help detect issues in stress levels and vulnerabilities that exist within those social configurations that could lead to further disruptions if left untreated and unchecked. Reaction techniques would include interventions that help regulate the child and family unit while they are going through a challenge. Recovery processes include repair ideas such as those noted in the earlier section on rupture and repair research as well as therapies and interventions that help people integrate and reconcile previous adverse experiences and conditions.

CHAPTER SUMMARY

In this chapter, we saw how guidelines and principles of systems resilience and engineering offer important parallels to how we can enhance our strategies for improving human communication, resilience, and optimized systems performance. As we keep in mind the above concepts of systems resilience, we will now briefly review some of the frameworks and ideas covered in previous chapters to give an outline of how these various perspectives come together into an overall understanding of human communication as it relates to regulation, attachment, and systems thinking.

BOOK SUMMARY

In Chapter 1, we explored the idea of systems, feedback, and what we are trying to do when we communicate. This includes the idea of systems thinking, which expands the space and time horizon to look at how the past interacts with the present and future trajectories, as well as all the interacting nodes and systems that influence each person's internal state, reactions, micro-gestures, behaviors, and intentions, as well as their anticipatory adjustments and expectations. We examined this through the lens of experience-dependent neuroplasticity and the building of brain architecture through attachment experiences and serve and return exchanges, particularly between mature brains and infant brains. Through that lens, we saw the relationship between social experiences, attunement, and responsiveness from caregivers and how this helps build circuitry in the brain to help process information and build autonomy and self-regulation.

In Chapter 2, our main focus was the concept of regulatory flexibility, and how flexibility itself is a strategy for resilience. We explored nonverbal components of communication within early attachment experiences and how the detection, processing, and expressing of vibrations and signals exchanged between caregiver and child correlate to the development of self-regulatory brain networks, particularly the orbital prefrontal cortex. The orbital prefrontal networks are involved in self-regulation, as well as procedural, memory, and socioaffective processes. They also relate to approach and avoidant behaviors and to the processing of facial expressions and selective attention to specific features of facial gestures, as well as visual and auditory inputs related to emotions. We integrated this into an understanding of self-regulation with the idea of regulatory flexibility, and the importance of developing context sensitivity, a repertoire of self-regulation strategies, and an ability to monitor and respond to feedback. These three pillars are important for expending energy adequately and appropriately to constantly emerging dynamics that occur in the environment and in interpersonal communication. Over-expenditure of energy relates to hyper-vigilance and detection of threat when it is not there or over-anticipation of reward that may become maladaptive. Inappropriate expenditures of energy toward threats and opportunities relate to the presence of unconscious filters and distorted cognitive processes, as well as attentional biases that are based particularly on past experiences. These rapid, initial appraisals involve implicit and procedural memory and activate ergotropic or trophotropic strategies within the nervous system. Ergotropic relates to energy expenditure and the sympathetic nervous system, while trophotropic relates to energy restoration and rest and the parasympathetic system. If events or conditions are not well matched to a person's neural and behavioral resources, the nervous system may become over-challenged and have difficulties in returning to baseline after a sympathetic or parasympathetic response, which can then lead to a chronic bias toward sympathetic or parasympathetic activity.

In Chapter 3, we looked at the importance of synchrony, attunement, and attachment and the interdependence of these within the realm of communication. We saw how communication—both verbal and nonverbal—is a biobehavioral attunement that supports affect synchrony. Affect synchrony includes autonomic reactivity, affiliative hormones, and brain activations and is also tied to vagal tone, heart rate coupling, and biological synchrony, which is influenced by voice, face, and micro behaviors. Within the framework of biological synchrony and communication as attunement to signals, we saw the important role of oxytocin and mammalian bonds. Oxytocin plays a role in stress reduction, enhances social competence, and is tied to optimal parenting, touch, and attunement. Lack of biobehavioral synchrony is associated with higher levels of cortisol and insecure attachment profiles. In adult relationships, we also see both nonverbal and verbal synchrony as related to vagal tone and oxytocin. High-risk parenting is related to a lack of biobehavioral synchrony and attunement and is associated with suboptimal outcomes within mental health and other forms of neural and psycho-social development.

In Chapter 4, the focus was primarily on communication as a behavioral transmitter and energy optimizer, particularly in the realm of survival, danger, and attachment. Communication is a tool for avoiding tissue damage danger as it acts as a warning signal, as well as a signal of the need for assistance and organized behavior against a threat. It is also an energy optimization tool as it functions as a sociobehavioral transmitter for human sociality, collective problem-solving, and nervous system regulation. We returned to the concept of attachment as a way for humans to use relationships to enhance vitality by regulating emotions and fear. Attachment is both a pattern of behavior, as well as a pattern of processing information, and it also serves as a strategy for identifying and responding to danger. In this chapter, we also explored the dynamic maturational model of human attachment as a response to danger, and that subcortical shortcuts are often used in response to danger. These shortcuts serve the purpose of fast reaction through mechanisms of omitting and distorting information. Although these can serve as protective strategies in childhood, they may form maladaptive strategies within future relationships across the lifespan. As communication is a relational tool to support life-enhancing strategies, distorted or maladaptive processing, and biases may result in suboptimal interactions and, therefore, degrade communication as a tool. This is why we continue to return to emotion regulation and related systems as a primary focus of communication.

The mechanics of signals, in particular facial expressions, was the focus of Chapter 5. Here we looked at emotion as a process that occurs in reaction to events in the environment, and how that reflects cognitive activity, physiological arousal, action tendencies, motor expression, and subjective feeling states. The muscular elements of facial configurations are driven by cumulated appraisals of events based on the relevance of the event, how events interact with goals, needs, and values, and a person's perceived ability to cope with the event and its consequences.

In Chapter 6, we turned our focus to voice-heart connections, and the relationship between voice and internal state, particularly as it relates to respiration. Acoustic parameters, such as frequency, pitch, loudness, quality, and prosody, are shown to show up differently in various conditions such as posttraumatic stress, anger, suicidality, depression, and sleep deprivation. These parameters also serve as informational cues for size, gender, and identity. We then looked at the Brunswikian Functional Lens model and saw that a producer of voice encodes various types of information, which then become distal cues that can be objectively measured. The receiver senses these distal cues using their auditory perceptual mechanisms and captures the signals, then makes judgments via a decoding or cue-utilization process. Successful communication occurs when the receiver accurately perceives and infers the information from cues sent by the producer. Fundamental frequency and energy distribution within the voice frequency spectrum play a role in representing the internal information of the producer, particularly as it relates to appraisals, such as having little control or coping potential over a situation. Relational dimensions also play a role in vocal prosody, emotional expression, and emotional language. These dimensions include dominance-nondominance, affection-hostility, involvement-detachment, composure-nervousness, and trust-distrust. Perceiving voice is a process of active listening that involves middle ear muscle modulations. Some mental health conditions present higher activation of certain brain regions linked with emotion and threat detection, such as the amygdala and insula, in response to louder or angrier voices compared with controls. The perception of prosody is also affected by some mental health conditions like schizophrenia, depression, and posttraumatic stress, and we see here that both the production and perception of voice are affected by various internal processes that may distort or enhance certain features in ways that make each person, perception and processing of voices, unique to their own histories and resources.

Chapter 7 explored nonverbal and verbal communication within the framework of social communication and the various components related to that framework, including sociocognitive factors like executive functioning and socioemotional factors like emotional regulation and sociolinguistic skills. All of these factors are interrelated with language abilities and also have strong associations with private speech and inner dialogue, which is mediated by attachment, relationships, and joint attention. Joint attention includes face-to-face interactions, vocalizations, and eye contact and is considered to form primary intersubjectivity. This forms the groundwork for secondary subjectivity, which is where attention becomes joined to an external, third entity. Joint attention is mutually reinforcing feedback that supports the development of neural networks for social cognition and language development. Attachment and joint attention are empirically linked: insecure attachment profiles reflect less face-to-face interactions and less coordination of joint attention. Joint attention and language have also been linked to the unique human cognitive feature of shared intentionality. This is the idea that humans view others as intentional agents. This cognitive feature forms the basis of awareness of one's own internal environment, as well as feedback from others to help us understand objects and people. This internal awareness and awareness of others forms the foundation of theory of mind (which can also be called social understanding). Both attunement and theory of mind are critical for developing language and communication abilities. The ability of a caregiver to respond to joint attention with their child is associated with the child's ability to acquire vocabulary. Mentalizing is another feature associated with theory of mind and verbal communication. It is the ability to identify and verbalize the mental and emotional states of others. Early experiences with others who are able to mentalize influence a child's language and emotion regulation abilities.

In Chapter 7, we also looked at emotional granularity as the ability to nuance and verbalize sensory and visceral information. The ability to put sensory experiences and autonomic arousal into words is an important component of emotional regulation. Studies on alexithymia find that people who have a harder time creating a referential link between the subsymbolic and symbolic processes may have challenges in requesting support from others and regulating their own emotions. This is potentially because sensory and autonomic experiences need a specific image within the nonverbal domain before they can be linked with words in the verbal domain. In contrast to concrete objects in our environment, which already have an image, emotions are abstractions and therefore need an extra process to create this image-link. This makes feelings much harder to verbalize than observable behaviors, features, or objects. When this feeling-image-word referential process does not happen, it may be an indicator that the autonomic arousal and sensory experiences that are occurring for a person are not followed by specific cognitive processes that play a role in emotion regulation. This lack of cognitive processing may lead to challenges in emotion regulation.

Chapter 8 focuses on maturity and executive functioning and the relationship between this and language as a cognitive niche. A cognitive niche is a thought-enabling, cognition-enhancing, animal-built structure that helps materialize thought into a physical presence of sounds in the air or words on a page. This cognitive niche helps us build executive functioning and complex perspective-taking. Linguistic abilities are highly influenced by social experience and are initially shared with others, then reformulated and developed into other higher-order mental capacities. Linguistic abilities are impacted by private and inner speech, which is influenced by the speech that surrounds each person, particularly when they are young. Research shows that verbally labeling tasks can enhance performance and problem-solving. We also looked at other components of language, such as relational frame theory. This theory proposes that schemas and many associations between stimuli and networks can induce responses based on only one of those factors within an associative network, even if the other stimuli are not present. This also relates to Lang's fear network, which proposes that we may engage in a fear response based only on associations that come from learned or deduced observations of others without a previous direct experience of that stimulus. We also saw that generic language plays a role in how we attribute traits to entire categories of people, and how generic, as opposed to nongeneric or individuated language can lead people to believe that certain features are inherently essential to a category of people rather than due to specific actions or behaviors of an individual.

Chapter 9 returned to the idea of systems thinking, and in particular systems resilience and systems engineering as foundations for understanding the role communication plays in survivability. We looked at survivability from a military definition of retaining mission-critical capabilities. As we explored in previous chapters, we saw that communication is a form of enhancing homeostasis which includes survival and projection into the future. Systems resilience and systems engineering can be useful for looking at how we can frame the mission, critical components, and strategies for human communication. There are passive and active forms of resilience, which include anticipation resistance. Active strategies, including detection, reaction, and recovery. The qualities of a resilient system include adaptability, availability, maintainability, performance, and reliability.

REFERENCES

[ACKOFF1994]Ackoff, R. L. (1994). Systems thinking and thinking systems. *System Dynamics Review, 10*, 175–188.

[BRTIS2019] Brtis, J., and Mcevilley, M.. (2019). *Systems Engineering for Resilience*. Colorado Springs, CO: The MITRE Corporation.

[CARLSON2012] Carlson, J., Haffenden, R., Bassett, Gilbert, Buehring, W., Collins, M., Folga, Steve, Petit, Frederic, Phillips, J., Verner, D., and Whitfield, R. (2012). Resilience: Theory and Application. 10.2172/1044521.

[CHRISTENSEN1993] Christensen, A., and Pasch, L. (1993). The sequence of marital conflict: An analysis of seven phases of marital conflict in distressed and nondistressed couples. *Clinical Psychology Review, 13*, 3–14.

[EKMAN1978] Ekman, P., and Friesen, W. V. (1978). *Facial Action Coding System*. Palo Alto, CA: Consulting Psychologists Press.

[FIRESMITH2003] Donald G. Firesmith. *Common Concepts Underlying Safety, Security, and Survivability Engineering*, Technical Note CMU/SEI-2003-TN-033, Software Engineering Institute, Pittsburgh, Pennsylvania, December 2003.

[FIRESMITH2019] Firesmith, D. (2019, November 25). System resilience: What exactly is it?. Retrieved July 4, 2023, from *https://insights.sei.cmu.edu/blog/system-resilience-what-exactly-is-it/*.

[FIRESMITH2020] Firesmith, D. (2020, April 27). System Resilience Part 7: 16 Guiding Principles for System Resilience. Retrieved July 4, 2023, from *https://insights.sei.cmu.edu/blog/system-resilience-part-7-16-guiding-principles-for-system-resilience/*.

[FREDERICKSON2005] Fredrickson, B. L., and Branigan, C. (2005). Positive emotions broaden the scope of attention and thought–action repertoires. *Cognition and Emotion, 19*, 313–332. doi: 10.1080/02699930441000238

[GOTTMAN1993] Gottman, J. M. (1993). The roles of conflict engagement, escalation or avoidance in marital interaction: A longitudinal view of five types of couples. *Journal of Consulting and Clinical Psychology, 61*, 6–15.

[GOTTMAN1994] Gottman, J. M. (1994). *What Predicts Divorce: The Relationship Between Marital Processes and Marital Outcomes*. Hillsdale, NJ: Erlbaum.

[GOTTMAN1996] Gottman, J. M. McCoy, K., Coan, J., and Collier, H. (1996). the specific affect coding system (SPAFF) for observing emotional communication in marital and family interaction. In J. M. Gottman (ed.), *What Predicts Divorce? The Measures* (pp. 112–195). Mahwah NJ: Lawrence Erlbaum Associates.

[GOTTMAN1998] Gottman, J. M., Coan, J., Carrere, S., and Swanson, C. (1998). Predicting marital happiness and stability from newlywed interactions. *Journal of Marriage and the Family, 60*, 5–22.

[GOTTMAN2001] Gottman, J., Levenson, R., Woodin, E., (2001). Facial expressions during marital conflict. *Journal of Family Communication*, *1*(1), 37–57.

[GOTTMAN2015] John M. Gottman, Janice Driver, and Amber Tabares (2015). Repair During Marital Conflict in Newlyweds: How Couples Move from Attack–Defend to Collaboration, *Journal of Family Psychotherapy*, 26: 2, 85-108.

[HOSSEINI2016] Hosseini, S., Barker, K., and Ramirez-Marquez, J. E. (2016) A review of definitions and measures of system resilience, *Reliability Engineering & System Safety*, *145*, 47–61.

[JULIEN1989] Julien, D., Markman, H. J., and Lindahl, K. M. (1989). A comparison of a global and a macroanalytic coding system: Implications for future trends in studying interactions. *Behavioral Assessment*, *11*, 81–100.

[KROKOFF1989] Krokoff, L. J., Gottman, J. M., and Haas, S. D. (1989). Validation of rapid couples interaction scoring system. *Behavioral Assessment*, *11*, 65–79.

[MATTHEWS1996] Matthews, L. S., Wickrama, K. A. S., and Conger, R. D. (1996). Predicting marital instability from spouse and observer reports of marital interaction. *Journal of Marriage and the Family*, 58, 641–655.

[SCHERER2013] Scherer, K. R., Mortillaro, M., and Mehu, M. (2013). Understanding the mechanisms underlying the production of facial expression of emotion: a componential perspective. *Emotion Review, 5*, 47–53. doi: 10.1177/1754073912451504

[SCHORE1994] Schore, A. (1994) *Affect Regulation and the Origin of the Self: The Neurobiology of Emotional Development*. Hillsdale, NJ: Erlbaum.

[WEISS1990] Weiss, R. L., and Tolman, A. O. (1990). The marital interaction coding system—global (MICS—G): A global companion to the MICS. *Behavioral Assessment*, *12*(3), 271–294.

*I*NDEX

A

Affect Regulation Scale (ARS), 168
Affect synchrony
    affiliative hormones and brain
        activation
        neuropeptide oxytocin (OT), 69
        salivary OT (sOT) levels, 70
    autonomic reactivity, 68
        and cardiac vagal tone, 68–69
Attachment experiences and brain
    development
    off-loading and outsourcing, 14–15
    orphanage scenario, 13
    serve and return feedback, 15–18
Attachment theory
    description of, 64
    secure *vs.* insecure attachment, 65
    self-regulation, 64
Attachment to a caregiver, 13

B

Biobehavioral synchrony, 66
    affect synchrony, 67 (*see also* Affect
        synchrony)
    bond formation, 67
    factors influencing, 74

high-risk parenting, 72–73
    lack of
        factors influencing, 74
        high-risk parenting, 72–73
    maternal synchrony, 67
    paternal synchrony, 67
    study of, 66
    verbal and nonverbal signals, 66
Biological shortcuts
    information processing errors, 92
    protective strategies, 94–97
    subcortical circuits, 94
    zone of proximal development
        (ZPD), 92

C

Cognitive flexibility and communication,
    201
Cognitive processes and distortions
    cognitive therapies, 205
    generic *vs.* nongeneric language,
        205–207
    Relational Frame Theory, 202
        and Lang Fear Network, 202–205
    self-disclosure and attributions,
        207–208

Communication
  behavioral transmitter, 87–88
  biobehavioral synchrony
    affect synchrony, 67
    bond formation, 67
    factors influencing, 74
    high-risk parenting, 72–73
    maternal synchrony, 67
    paternal synchrony, 67
    study of, 66
    verbal and nonverbal signals, 66
  definition, 1
  direct contact *vs.* telereception, 102
  effective mechanisms, 66
  feedback, stress regulation, and
    autonomic responses
    ergotropic and trophotropic,
      42–43
    inescapability, 44–45
    limited data, 48–50
    predictive biases, 45–48
    repetitive exposure, 45
  human voice mechanisms and
    features
    acoustic features of vocalizations,
      127–131
    affective state, 131–132
    source-filter theory, 126–127
    speech production, 131
    subglottal system, 125
    supralaryngeal vocal tract, 126
    vocal folds, 126
  modern attachment theory
    danger, adaptation, and
      maladaptation, 90–91
    disorganized attachment, 89
    dynamic-maturational model of
      attachment and adaptation
      (DMM), 89–90

    principles of, 89
    short cutting, 91–97
  movements and vibrations, 3
  nonhuman species, 2
  optimization, 84–86
    through sociality, 86–87
  role of eyes in
    eye gaze, 105–106
    pupil dilation, 104–105
  role of facial expressions
    component process model of
      emotion (CPM), 107–111
  for survival
    aspects of, 81
    complex adaptive system, 80
    feedback-response
      mechanism, 80
    tissue-damage danger, 81
  voice and, 122
    information contained in, 136–140
    perceiving sounds, 140–146
  voice-face-heart connection, 122–125
  voice features and mental health
    anger and cardiovascular
      reactivity, 136
    depression, 134–135
    post-traumatic stress disorder
      (PTSD), 136
    sleep deprivation, 136
    stress, 132–134
    suicidality, 135–136
  voluntary *vs.* involuntary systems,
    102–104
Communication-for-survival process,
  80–81
Component process model of emotion
  (CPM)
  categories of appraisal, 110
  Corrugator supercilii, 108

Frontalis, 109–110
zygomaticus major muscle, 109
Couples Interactions Scoring System
    (CISS), 225

D

Duchenne smile, 112–113
Dynamic-Maturational Model (DMM),
    94–97

E

Electroencephalography (EEG), 10
Electroreception, 102
Embodied cognition model, 111
Emotional Facial Action Coding System
    (EMFACS), 112
Emotional facial expression, effects of
    trauma on, 112–114
Experience-dependent
    development, 9–12
Experience-expectant
    development, 9

F

Feedback exchange
    contingent responsivity, 19–20
    face-to-face interactions, 18
    moment-to-moment analysis, 18–19

H

High-risk parenting, 72–73, 230, 234
Homeostasis, 84
    fallacy of uniform efficacy, 63
    flexibility, 63
    goal of, 62
    mission of, 229
    for resilience and system
        regulation, 79

I

Interoception, 104

L

Law of Retention, 141
Locomotion, 11, 20
    social referencing, 20–21

O

Oxytocin, 70
    bonding and reducing stress, 70
    gender-specific differences, 71

P

Perceptual symbols
    systems (PSS), 111
Primary intersubjectivity, 163
Psychosocial deprivation, 10

R

Regulation theory. *see* Attachment
    theory
Regulatory flexibility, 30
    challenges
        anticipation and preparation, 41
        declarative memory, 39
        implicit and procedural memory,
            38–39
        orbital prefrontal system, 39–41
    concept of, 31
    context sensitivity and insensitivity,
        32–33
    feedback, 34
        internal, 34–36
        responsiveness, 36–37
        social, 36
    repertoire, 33

Relational Frame Theory, 202
  derived relational responding, 204
  key principles of, 204
  and Lang Fear Network, 202–205

S

Social Communication (SoCom)
  components of, 162
  executive functioning, 162–163
  joint attention, 163–164
  language is a bridge
    alexithymia, 167–170
    emotional granularity, 166–167
    language superiority effect, 166
  nonverbal and verbal
      components, 165
    prioritization of emotional cues,
      170–176
  and social synchrony, 163
  Theory of Mind (ToM), 164
Social synchrony, 163. *see also*
    Biobehavorial synchrony
Social understanding (SU)
  and language
    cognitive niche, 198
    executive functioning, 199
    psychological tool, 198
    social-context input, 197
  private and inner speech, 199–201
  theories, 196
Stimulus-Organism-Response model, 8
Systems resilience
  adverse events, 219
    active and passive resilience,
      220–221
  assets
    system components, 227
    system data, 227
    system-external assets, 227–228

flexible responsiveness, 224
guiding principles
  anticipate, resist, detect, react,
    recover, 231
  anticipation and resistance, 231
  common critical assets,
    concentrate on, 229–230
  critical assets identification, 229
  detection, reaction, recovery,
    231–232
  disruptive harm, concentrate on,
    230
  expect and identify adversities,
    230
  mission-critical capabilities, focus
    on, 229
protection
  detection techniques, 222–223
  reactions, 223
  recovery, 223–224
  resistance, 221
quality attributes, 228–229
rupture and repair strategies, 225
and survivability, 216–218
Systems thinking, 61
  complexity, 7
  control mechanisms, 8
  emergent, 5
  energy-conservation perspective, 7
  fundamental aspect of, 4
  sensory receptors, 8
  stimulus-response paradigm, 6
  time and space, 5–6

T

Telereception, 102
Tissue-damage danger
  organize behavior for threat-
    prevention, 83–84

prevent proximity of a threat, 82
request proximity of a source of
    support, 82–83
Toronto Alexithymia Scale (TAS), 167

V

Voice and communication, 122
    features and mental health
        anger and cardiovascular
            reactivity, 136
        depression, 134–135
        post-traumatic stress disorder
            (PTSD), 136
        sleep deprivation, 136
        stress, 132–134
        suicidality, 135–136
    information contained in
        affection-hostility, 139
        aspects of, 137

Brunswikian functional lens
    model, 137
composure-nervousness, 139
dominance-non-dominance, 139
energy distribution in the
    spectrum, 138
fundamental frequency, 138
involvement-detachment, 139
mean energy, 138
trust-distrust, 139–140
voice production and reception,
    140
perceiving sounds
    middle ear, physiology of, 142–145
    positive emotions, 146
    Social Anxiety Disorder (SAD),
        145
    sound frequencies and nervous
        system responses, 141–142
voice-face-heart connection, 122–125

www.ingramcontent.com/pod-product-compliance
Lightning Source LLC
Chambersburg PA
CBHW061359210326
41598CB00035B/6029